Natural Birth:
The Power of the Woman's Body

A guide for first time mamas

2nd edition

Sandra Lena

ISBN: 979-8-86808680-9 (hbk)
ISBN: 979-8-87117776-1 (pbk)
ISBN: 979-8-86808829-2 (pbk)

To my son and to all women
seeking a positive birth experience.

We all have doubts, even when
we trained ourselves to be prepared.
Remember you are the best person
to give birth to your baby.
You can and you will.

Contents

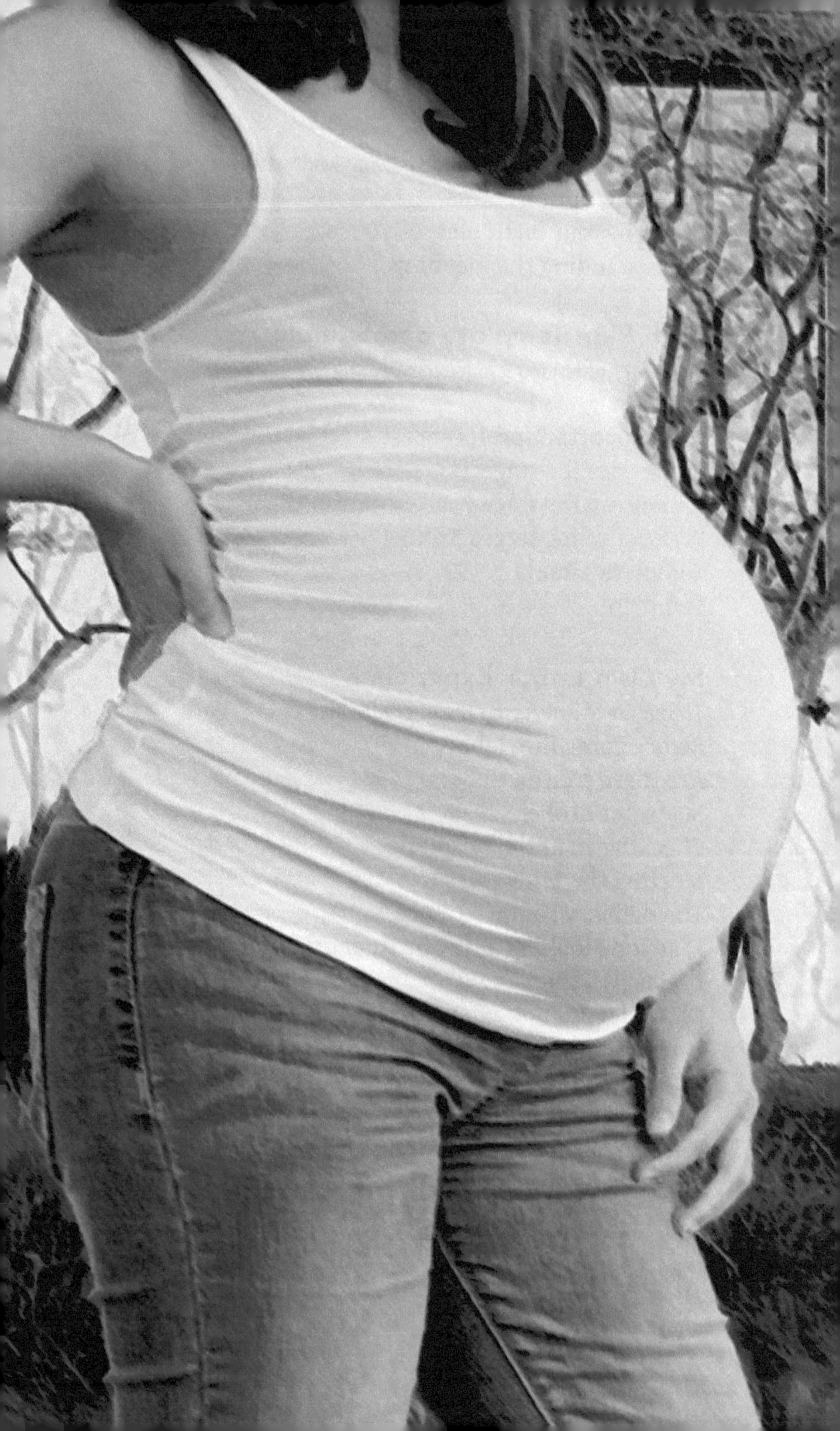

Introduction

During my pregnancy, I read tons of books, took many pregnancy courses, listened to podcasts, and watched plenty of videos from *doulas*, midwives and medical personnel. I exposed myself to different points of view. I wanted to be as prepared as possible. After all, for many of us, giving birth is one of the most important and magical moments of our life. An athlete trains intensively for months to run a marathon that on the day will take 4-5 hours to finish. A student prepares for years to obtain a degree. A birth can go anywhere from a few hours to over a day. Why not do the same for the birth of our child? Be informed and nurture our mind and body to have the birth we want?

I am a certified prenatal and postnatal fitness instructor and throughout this pregnancy I have learned even more about me, my body, and my mind . Everything I feel and experience, the baby does too. One night, I was exhausted after a very long day of running errands and finishing a loaded work day. I was also stressed out. That day, from the inside out, I felt something I had never felt before; it was painful in a way I cannot describe. That was my baby telling me, "that's enough." I stopped everything, took a seat, and closed my eyes. I connected to myself and my baby, and I calmed myself down. At that moment, I learned this is not just me anymore.

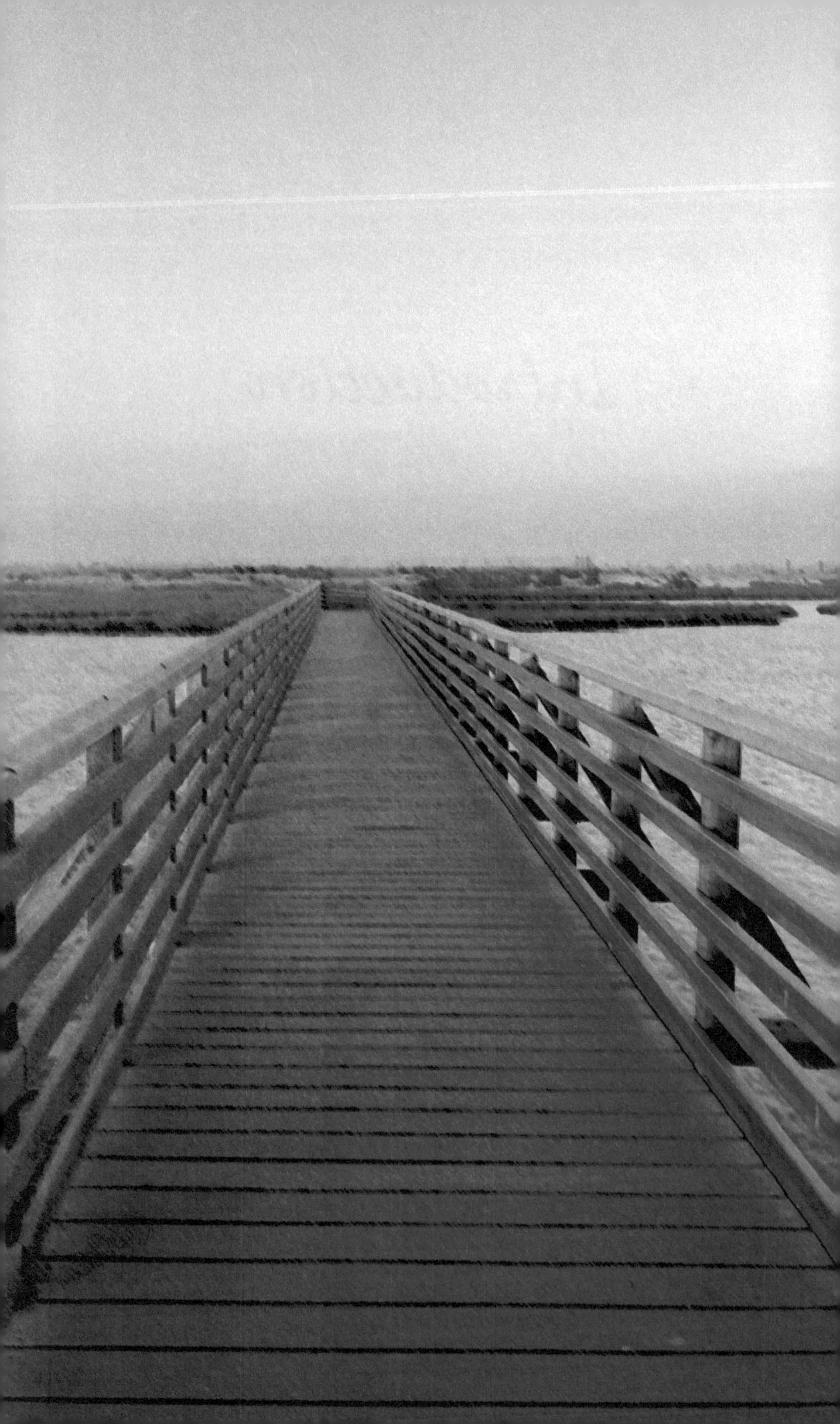

Pregnancy Prep

*The power of mental and physical exercises
to get our mind and body ready*

At the moment of giving birth, our body and mind experience one of the most intense moments they will ever go through. There is power in feeling prepared. To many women, the labor process brings doubt and uncertainty. Preparing ourselves mentally and physically will allow us to avoid those distractions and focus on the birth. Our future selves will thank us for it.

Meditation is the bedrock of pregnancy preparation. It can be surprising how well it works. Once we are able to concentrate on meditating, we feel completely differently. It has so many benefits: positivity, serenity, relaxation, and empowerment. Meditating can be hard because unrelated thoughts often come through. The moment we let them pass by, however, we can sense and feel the true benefits of meditation.

Physical exercises are a great tool to prepare our body for the level of effort and resilience birth requires. It is important to find balance. Sitting down and/or laying down all day throughout the pregnancy will most likely cause our muscles and ligaments to atrophy or get swollen. At the same time, excessive exercise can be counterproductive. As the pregnancy progresses, our body experiences changes and, even when exercising often, our ability to do certain movements will decrease and we will need to adapt. It is okay to stay active as long as we listen to our body and adjust our workouts accordingly.

Meditation & Visualization

Nurturing and nourish our mind is essential. Meditating is training our mind in awareness to get a healthy sense of calm and perspective. When we meditate, we work on the ability to stay focused, which allows us to be present and fully engaged in the now. Likewise, visualizing consists of picturing someone or something—even an experience—through our imagination. This mind tool brings us a sense of warmth and ease creating a safe space aside from distractions.

Acceptance meditation

As we familiarize ourselves with how we feel, we widen our capacity to live with those feelings. The more we clue into ourselves with what we feel, the more flexible our minds become.

At first, it's easy for many moms to think over pregnancy and birth experiences. Stories someone told us, or we read. However, the key is to allow ourselves to be okay with our own feelings. The goal is to connect with what we are feeling with honesty. Diverse experiences and thoughts will evoke different feelings and that is good.

Now, we are going to put a pause to our thinking selves and let our minds rest. We adjust our posture to feel comfortable. We allow our body to soften onto the chair or floor beneath us. We close our eyes. Then, we inhale and exhale at our own pace. Little by little, we make the inhales deeper and the exhales longer.

- We relax and settle into the space.
- We notice the sounds around us.
- We bring the focus back to the body and notice if we feel light or heavy.

- We scan down the body, from the head to the feet, acknowledging every part.
- We want to connect to the sense of purpose. What is my motivation? Why am I meditating?
- How do I feel right now?
- I soften the eyebrows and relax the jaw.
- Focusing back on our body, we pay attention to how it moves up and down with every inhale and exhale.
- Accepting my feelings as I inhale, embracing the thoughts to keep and letting go of unneeded thoughts as I exhale.

I open my eyes and start waking up my body. Gently, I move my head, my shoulders, my arms, the tips of my fingers, my legs, my feet and my toes.

Grateful meditation

The principle of this meditation is to show gratitude to our body for its work during our pregnancy journey. For this meditation, we get ourselves in a comfortable position and close our eyes. We breathe in and out, slowly. We are going to focus on three crucial parts of our body and thank them for the amazing work it does.

- We focus on our feet. Are they touching the ground? Are they cold or hot? Are they bare and free or do they have socks on? Are my toes moving?
- I love me feet, and I am grateful because they are keeping strong letting me go places.
- We focus on our legs. Are they extended or bent? Are they cold or hot? Do they feel any pressure? What happens if I wiggle them?
- I love my legs, and I am grateful because they are supporting my changing body.
- We focus on our belly. What month am I in? Do I sense my baby yet? Is my skin soft? What do I feel when I place my hands on it?
- I love my belly, and I am grateful because it is growing my beloved baby.

Deep belly meditation and visualization

We sit down on a chair, couch, or yoga mat. We cross our legs in the lotus position. We place our hands on our belly, gently cradling our baby bump, and breathe slowly, at our own pace—in and out. We observe the sensations we feel beneath our hands and focus our thoughts on them. Is my baby moving? Is my baby calm with me now? Do I feel warmth? Is my skin soft? As we go through the different questions, we allow ourselves to think about the answers to each question in our own time.

Then, we visualize our baby and allow time to really connect with each image.

- We visualize our baby being happy, enjoying their time in the womb, moving around their tiny little hands and tiny little feet.
- We visualize our baby safe and protected by the amniotic fluid and the uterus.
- We visualize our baby knowing where to go when the time comes.
- We visualize ourselves knowing what to do to help them have the most amazing experience at birth.

We allow all thoughts related to our baby and us, and disregard unwanted thoughts, letting them pass by.

Uterus visualization

The uterus is connected to our emotions and thoughts. Bringing positive thoughts when visualizing the uterus encourages our body to produce endorphins and serotonin. This modulates our mood and takes the pain away.

On a floor mat or the bed, we lay back. We can add a cushion under our lower back for support. We put our knees up and our legs on the mat. We place our hands on our belly, below our belly button. We close our eyes, loosen our forehead and relax our mouth, leaving it semi-open. Now we breathe deeply three or four times focusing on the movement of our belly as we inhale and exhale. The goal is to reach calmness and relaxation.

- We smile and visualize that smile in and out, we feel how smiling brings happiness and relaxation to our whole body.
- We focus on our uterus. With each inhale and exhale, we visualize the uterus moving, expanding, and relaxing.

As we continue breathing, we allow ourselves to give our uterus the importance it deserves. Our uterus is full of vitality. Our uterus is capable of creating life. The uterus is, with the heart, the strongest muscle in our body.

- Then, we visualize our pelvic area and perineal muscles. We imagine them expanding and relaxing. Getting thinner and softer. Becoming elastic.
- We welcome our emotions without judging and let unrelated thoughts pass by.

Finally, we breathe deeply three times, open our eyes, and allow our body to stretch. Then, we prop ourselves up slowly.

Ocean visualization

During contractions, we can help decrease the intensity of pain using visualization. As we practice for our labor, we visualize the waves in the ocean.

We sit down on a chair, couch, or yoga mat. We cross our legs in the lotus position. We inhale through our nose as we expand our diaphragm and exhale through our mouth releasing the air at our own pace.

While we breathe, we visualize the ocean and mentally imagine each contraction as a wave.

- We watch each wave slowly peak in intensity. Then, we allow each wave to slowly come down.
- The focus is not on the peak but after the peak.
- The focus is where the ocean comes back to calm, and recovers its strength to go again.

There is always calm after the peak. After the wave rises, the water always comes back down. That is where our focus should be.

To help keep our focus, we can imagine ourselves as a jellyfish, allowing the waves to wash through us. Letting ourselves go and move with the ocean.

Physical prep

Hip rotations

We can do this type of pregnancy fitness on a birthing ball or yoga ball. Alternatively, we can do it on the floor, or on top of a yoga mat.

Using a ball: We sit down on a yoga ball and do rotations with our hips. We can start by doing 10 repetitions in each direction. After that, we increase the number of repetitions to reach two minutes of hip rotation to one side. Then, we do two minutes of rotation to the other side.

Using a mat: We put our hands and knees on the mat and do the same hip rotations.

Hip straight-line moments

We can do this type of pregnancy fitness on a birthing ball or yoga ball. Alternatively, we can do it on the floor, or on top of a yoga mat.

Using a ball: We sit down on a yoga ball and do straight-line movements with our hips. We can start by doing 10 repetitions in each direction. After that, we increase the number of repetitions to get to two minutes for each movement. There are three types of line movements.

- Front to back
- Side to side
- Diagonal

Using a mat: We put our hands and knees on the mat and do the same hip straight-line movements.

U hip movements

We can do this type of pregnancy fitness on a birthing ball or yoga ball. Alternatively, we can do it on the floor, or on top of a yoga mat.

Using a ball: We sit down on a yoga ball and do U movements with our hips. We move our hips as much forward and to the right as we can. We start drawing a U with our hips going back to the center of the ball. Then, we move the hips to the front and left. After that, back and center again. Finally, forward and to the right. We can start by doing 10 repetitions and increasing the number of repetitions to get to two minutes.

Using a mat: We put our hands and knees on the mat and do the same U hip movements.

"Bouncy, bouncy"

On a yoga ball, we sit down and bounce on it, freely but carefully. This is a great way to release tension at the same time we work our pelvic floor.

We can start by doing 20-30 repetitions After that, we increase the number of repetitions to get to two minutes.

"Walking" on a chair

For this exercise, we sit down on a chair. We place our behinds on the very back of the chair and we inch forward moving one glute at a time, as if we were walking with our backside. We go all the way to the end of the chair. Depending on the chair, it takes about six movements to reach the end of the chair. Then, we do the same going backward.

We repeat this exercise six to ten times.

Extended leg stretches

On a yoga mat: We lay down on our side with our legs extended and a little forward so our toes are passed our hips.

- We inhale as we lift one of our legs up.
- We exhale as we bring our other leg down.

We do 3 series of 8 repetitions per each side.

Circle leg stretches

On a yoga mat: We lay down on our side with our legs on a 90 degree-angle from our hips to our knees and 90 degrees from our knees to our ankles. Like if we would be on a chair. Now, we draw circles with the knee of our top leg and breathe as we need to.

We do 3 series of 8 repetitions per each side.

Open up hip and leg stretches

On a yoga mat: We lay down on our side with our legs on a 90 degree-angle from our hips to our knees and 90 degrees from our knees to our ankles. Like if we would be on a chair. Now, starting the movement with the knees, we move them up and down, as if we were opening and closing a book. For this exercise, we can alternate legs, or workout both at the same time.

- We inhale as one of our knees moves down and to the side.
- We exhale as our other knee moves up and to the center.

We do 3 series of 8 repetitions per each side.

Rocking technique

On a mat: We put our hands and knees on the mat. We rock front and back alternating our knees and ankles' position. This technique will be crucial and advantageous during labor.

- Knees out, ankles in to help open the upper part of the pelvis as baby starts descending.
- Knees in, ankles out to help open the lower part of the pelvis as baby is ready to get out.

Wiggle the tail

On a mat: We put our hands and knees on the mat. We move the end part of our back, where our coccyx bone is like a dog would move his tail. A great exercise to relax the end of our back, especially for sciatica pain.

Cat/Cow movements

On a mat: We put our hands and knees on the mat. We arch our back in and out. A basic motion that can be enormously beneficial in supporting the back and easing pain. These movements are one of the most stress-relieving and calming in the early stage of labor.
- We inhale as we tilt our pelvis back for cow pose.
- We exhale as we tuck our tailbone for cat pose.

Frog movements

On a mat: We put our hands and knees on the mat. With our knees spread wide and our feet close to each other, we extend our arms in front of us. Then, we put our body all the way back, having our tailbone touch our feet if possible. Then, all the way forward like a frog about to jump would do. These movements are one of the most stress-relieving and calming in the early stage of labor.
- Inhale as we retract our body all the way back.
- Exhale as we extend our body all the way forward.

Physical prep with partner

Wiggles

This is a great exercise for releasing tension, and it consists of two parts.

First: On a yoga mat, we place our hands and knees down, and our partner stands behind us. They place their hands on our hips and gently move them to massage the muscles around our hips and pelvic area.

Second: Our partner then works on our legs, starting from the top and moving down to our knees. If we have swollen feet or legs (pregnancy edema), our partner can continue down to our ankles and back up to the top of our legs. For this second part, we have a few position options:

- We can maintain the same position with our hands and knees on the mat.
- We can lie on our backs while propping ourselves up slightly with our elbows on the mat.
- We can lie on our backs and place a pillow at the end of our back for support (note that it is not recommended for pregnant women to lie flat on their backs, especially for extended periods).

Counter-Pressure

We can choose from any position that makes us feel comfortable, but the most common options are these three:

- Leaning forward on a chair (optionally with a pillow on top for added comfort).
- Resting on our yoga ball with our knees on the floor and our head and elbows on the ball.
- Putting our hands and knees on a floor mat.

Our partner stands behind us, facing our back. Using both hands, they apply a steady, firm force first to our lower back and then to the side of each hip. They can apply and release pressure in 10-15 second intervals for 2-3 minutes.

Rebozo

A rebozo is a shawl. The rebozo technique involves using a shawl to provide support and relieve pressure from our bodies, especially our growing pregnant belly. There are three great exercises for using the rebozo or shawl.

- In the first one, either our partner or we fold the shawl lengthwise and wrap it somewhat tightly under our belly and hips. Our partner stands behind us, facing our back. Then, by grabbing the ends of

the shawl, our partner pulls gently. The tightness
of the shawl offers support and stability. Towards
the end of pregnancy, it is extremely useful to helps
alleviate the weight of the heavy belly.
- For the second exercise, in the same position, our
partner gently moves their hands back and forth to
create a soothing sensation around the belly.
- In the third exercise, we place the rebozo around our
lower back and hips while facing our partner. Our
partner takes hold of the two ends of the rebozo. We
slowly lower ourselves into a squat, ensuring that
our partner supports us to prevent losing balance.

Reflexology

During pregnancy, reflexology aims to optimize the
physical and emotional health of the pregnant woman, and
it can be effective in alleviating issues such as low back pain,
heartburn, anxiety, and depression.

When focusing on the hands, our partner uses their
thumb to apply gentle pressure to the lower side of our palms,
right at the edge between our palm and wrist. They move their
thumb in a C-shaped motion from one side of the lower palm to
the other, sometimes extending all the way up to the thumb of
our hand. (Refer to the image below.)

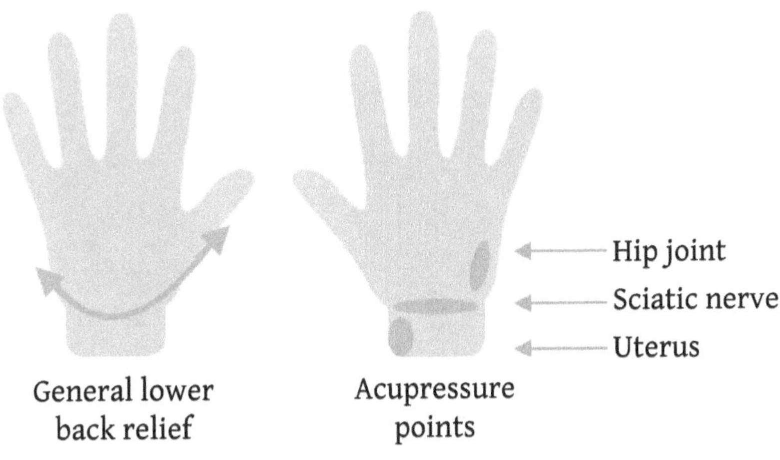

General lower
back relief

Acupressure
points

For the feet, our partner uses their thumb to apply gentle pressure to specific key acupressure points on our foot and moves their thumb in various directions. (Refer to the image below.)

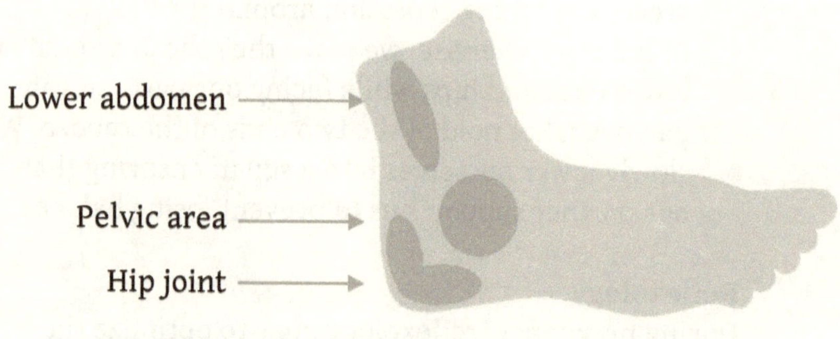

In our feet, we have various acupressure points that can help relieve the same parts of our body. Working on all these different points can further alleviate that particular area to an even greater extent.

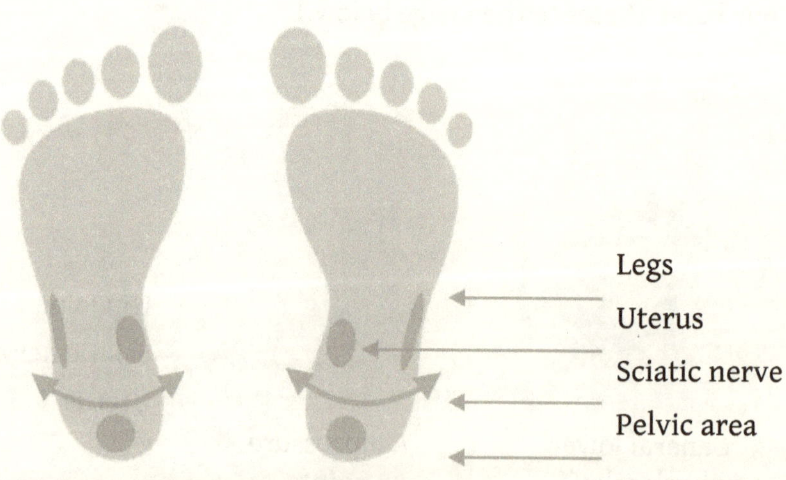

Massage

Massages are an excellent way to relax our minds and muscles, especially during pregnancy. They help release stress and tension, leaving us feeling balanced and energized. Additionally, dimming the lights and playing some soothing instrumental music can significantly enhance the relaxation experience.

When it comes to massages, we have several options:

- Laying forward on a chair (with a pillow at the top for added comfort).
- Resting on our yoga ball with our knees on the floor and our head and elbows on the ball.
- Positioning ourselves on a floor mat with our knees and hands.

Our partner can begin with a gentle massage focusing on the lower back. Then, they can work on our legs all the way down to our feet. This second part is particularly beneficial on days when our legs or feet are swollen. Finally, a gentle massage around the neck area can be very soothing.

Perineal Massage

The perineal massage is a gentle, manual stretching of our pelvic floor. This massage helps prepare the muscles and skin between our vagina and rectum for childbirth. While the idea of perineal massage may initially seem unusual or intimidating, the positive benefits make it well worth trying. Moreover, the awkwardness tends to diminish after the first attempt.

Starting around week 32, we should plan to repeat this massage twice a week, or even daily, until delivery. After giving birth, perineal massages are no longer necessary and can, in fact, be uncomfortable. Instead, we can transition to doing *Kegel* exercises, which involve gentle pelvic floor contractions. Regular *Kegels* can help with pelvic floor dysfunction, pain, or incontinence.

The benefits of perineal massage are significant. It reduces the risk of tearing or experiencing high-degree tears. It also brings down the risk of having an *episiotomy*, a surgical cut between the vagina and rectum. We can perform this massage by ourself, have our partner assist us, or use a *Perimom*, a perineal massage tool designed to help reach and massage the perineum area.

To get started, we should thoroughly wash our hands (and trim our nails). We sit in a relaxed position with our legs bent and our knees spread wide. Apply a few drops of olive oil, almond oil, or coconut oil to our perineum and thumb. For the massage, we gently insert our thumb at the bottom of the vaginal wall and apply gentle pressure downward, toward our rectum.

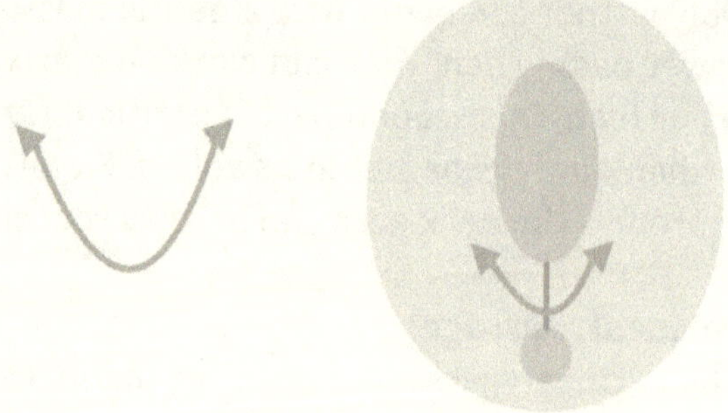

Maintain the pressure and move our thumb from left to right in a U-shaped pattern (from about 3 to 9 o'clock). We can do this for 3-5 minutes. It's normal to feel a stretch and a bit of stinging or burning, but we should never experience pain.

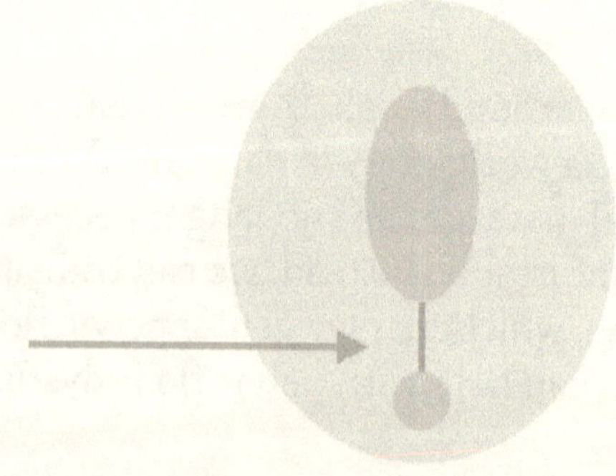

Next, perform three careful stretches. We repeat each stretch three times, holding each one for 15 to 45 seconds. We can increase the holding time with each stretch. We need to remember that the goal of this exercises is to help us during the delivery of our baby. We should feel comfortable.

- The first stretch is downward.
- The second is downward and diagonally to the left
- The third is downward and diagonally to the right.

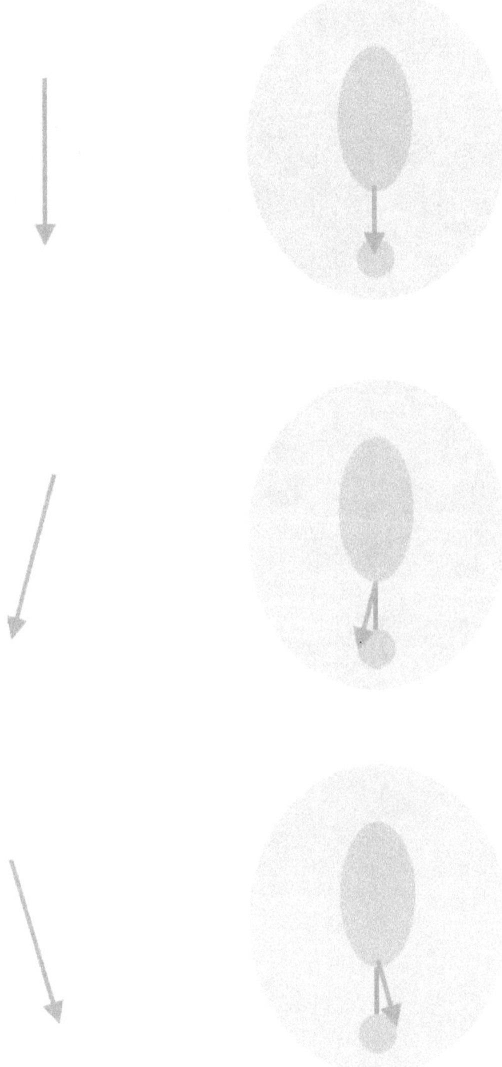

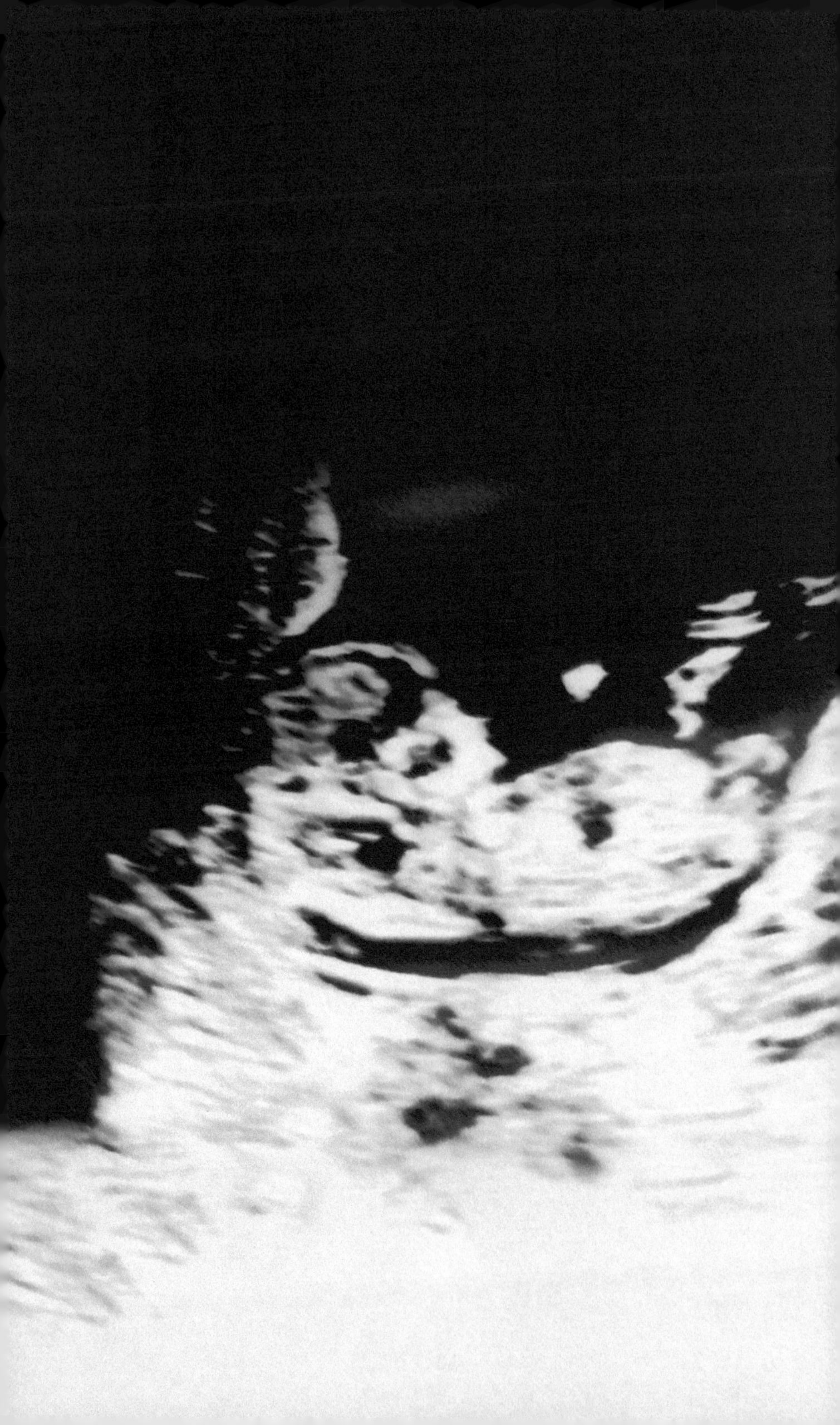

Labor Stages

*The power of understanding
each stage and its patterns*

Thinking about going into labor can be frustrating and confusing, but it doesn't have to be that way. By knowing what to expect and how to identify each stage of labor, we can manage our stress levels and expectations.

First stage

The first stage consists of three parts:

Early labor
Usually the longest stage. However, every woman is different, and no two labors are the same. As a guide, it can last anywhere from a few hours to over a day. A way to identify we are in labor is when our contractions last about 30-45 seconds.

Some ways (or tricks) to know we are in labor or that labor is imminent:
- Losing our mucus plug (also called bloody show): this means the cervix is changing to prepare for delivery. The mucus plug is a vaginal discharge that has a

viscous-like texture; it can be transparent, pink, or bloody. When the mucus plug is completely clear, labor can still be days or weeks away. When it has a more pink or brown bloody tint, it normally means labor is about to start within the next hour or or in up to two days. If the discharge becomes bright red, it is recommended to call the practitioner right away.

- Rupture of membranes, better known as "my water just broke": it is usually a fluid with a clear or pink-tinted color that feels like a gush or steady trickle from the vagina. Once the water breaks, labor normally will start within 12-24 hours, but it can also start right away. However, some women do not notice their water breaking, and most women do not break water until they are well into labor.

When the water breaks it is important to note what some refer to as the *TACO* information. We must remember it tell it to our nurse, doctor, or midwife when they ask us.

TIME: when it broke
AMOUNT: how much liquid
COLOR: it should be transparent/close to no color
ODOR: no smell is good

It is hard to know how dilated we are without the help of a medical professional or midwife, but the cervix dilates to about 3-4 cm at this point.

Contractions have a pattern, typically starting with one or two per hour. They will not go away (like they did with the Braxton Hicks contractions) and will gradually get stronger and more frequent (getting to about 10 minutes between contractions).

- Braxton Hicks are practice contractions. It is when our uterus contracts to get our body ready for labor. These Braxton Hicks contractions are irregular and go away after having one, or a few.

We can continue to go about our day. We will keep a mild activity level, stay hydrated, and eat if we feel hungry. To start on the right foot, we will also try to rest, stretch, sit on the birth ball, change positions, or even soak in the tub. It is important to keep relaxed and manage any possible pain as contractions increase.

We will start timing our contractions to know how far apart they are and how long each one lasts. There are many useful apps that we can set in our phones (before labor day) to help us in this task.

> 5-1-1: A general rule of thumb is to head to the hospital if the contractions are five minutes apart, lasting one minute long for at least one hour.

Active labor
Every woman is different, but, in general, active labor can last about three to five hours with contractions increasing in frequency and lasting about 60 seconds.

The cervix can start dilating more quickly from about 3-4 cm to 7 cm.

Contractions will get intense and will command our attention. If our water didn't break before, it might break now, making the contractions speed up. It is important to continue any relaxation techniques and coping mechanisms that make us feel comfortable. During the rest period in between contractions, it is especially crucial to maintain relaxation because it saves our energy and helps our cervix open.

Transition phase

This is usually the shortest stage, lasting anywhere from a few minutes to a couple of hours, and contractions can last 60-90 seconds with only 30 seconds to two minutes in between.

The contractions get very intense during this phase and cause a strong feeling of pressure in the lower back for many women. There is very little time to rest, and we might feel tired, hot and cold in a matter of seconds, and perhaps frustrated. This is normal, and we can let these feelings pass by focusing on our baby being almost with us.

INHALE/EXHALE: Breathe, breathe, breathe
VISUALIZATIONS: Ocean visualization
CHANGE POSITIONS: As much as you need

Breathing exercises are crucial at this point. We will change positions as needed to ease pain, and ask for help if we need it. Having positive encouragement and companionship has a big impact on how we feel during this stage.

Second stage

Aside of the dilation and effacement (thinning) of the cervix, doctors measure the fetal station of the baby. This is a measure on a scale from -5 to +5 or -3 to +3 (depending on the doctor), and it looks like this:

-5 to 0	Floating station: The most palpable part of the baby is above the ischial spines.
zero station	Engage station: The baby's head is "engaged," or aligned with the ischial spines.
0 to +5	The baby has descended beyond the ischial spines.

Pushing

Pushing can last anywhere from 20 minutes to a couple of hours, and the contractions can move a little further apart to allow longer rest periods in between each one.

This stage starts once our cervix is at 10 cm—that is as wide open as it needs to be.

We might want to labor down:
- When we labor down we hold for the involuntary muscle that is our uterus to start the work of pushing.
- This will help reduce the risk of tearing.
- Our cervix is fully dilated, but the skin around the area and our perineum (the tissue between our vagina and rectum) might be a little tense.
- By laboring down and waiting to feel the urge to push, we allow our bodies to get completely ready, which reduces the risk of tears and conserves our body's energy.

The urge to push:
- It might feel a lot like needing to go #2, and this might actually happen, which is perfectly normal and expected.

The ring of fire:
- We might feel a burning or stinging sensation.
- It happens during crowning.
- The feeling is a more intense version of the heat felt sometimes during preparation with perineal massages (explained in the Pregnancy Prep Chapter).

The strong feelings we experience during this stage of childbirth are why it is crucial to do mental and physical exercises during pregnancy. Is in this moment when we really thank ourselves for all the preparation.

Pushing can be both the most challenging and the most rewarding part of the process. With each push, we bring the baby closer and closer. Once the baby begins crowning, we're just a few more pushes away from the finish line. Pushing is a unique and remarkable experience, just moments away of the happiness of meeting our newborn baby.

Delivery of the baby
All that hard work has finally paid off. Our baby is with us. We've just gone through many hours of intense mental and physical work, and we might feel exhausted. However, as soon as we see our baby for the first time, any uncomfortable feelings will vanish. Our baby might look a bit unusual at first, with some blood on their head, and their head may appear somewhat cone-shaped, but as long as everything is well, we will be holding our precious little one in a matter of seconds. In the event that something requires checking or if there are any concerns, the nurses will attend to the baby (whether in the same room or a different one; in which case, the father/partner can accompany them). Later, they will place the baby on our chest.

Cord clamping:
- Cutting the umbilical cord.
- It is best to cut the cord once the pulsing has slowed down or stopped, this gives time for the baby to adapt to the new environment and the new type of breathing. This takes about 45-60 seconds.
- If donating the cord blood or putting it in a private cord blood bank, the cord will need to be cut while it is still pulsing.

Vernix:
- The vernix is a creamy, white covering on the baby.
- The amount of vernix left on the skin at birth varies widely depending on how much of it got absorbed before birth.
- When the vernix is present, the WHO (World Health Organization) recommends leaving it on the baby for his/her skin to absorb it.
- The vernix warms the baby's body and stabilizes their blood sugar levels. It also acts as an antibacterial barrier, helping the baby adapt to their new surroundings and giving their immune system time to strengthen.

Golden hour:
- The very first hour of a baby's life is key, as they start to adapt to the new environment.
- Skin-to-skin contact is a top priority during this time.

Skin-to-skin:
- It benefits the baby as it helps regulate the baby's temperature, breathing, and heart rate.
- It also benefits the mother experiencing the bond with the baby, reducing stress hormones, and even encouraging early latching.

Breastfeeding:
- Right after birth and for a few days, mom's body produces *colostrum,* a thick and usually golden-yellow breast-milk that has all of the nutrients and antibodies the baby needs.
- Most full-term babies are ready and eager to start breastfeeding within 30 min-2 hours after birth. Nevertheless, after that first feeding, the baby might not be very hungry for the next day to day and a half.

Third stage

Delivery of the placenta
This stage can last 5-30 minutes, depending on the birthing mother.

It takes a few more contractions for the placenta to separate from the uterine wall. Pushing during these last contractions can help things progress. Sometimes, the nurses might also apply pressure or knead the abdomen to assist in the detachment.

Delivering the placenta can be barely noticeable or might cause some discomfort or pain. At this point, we and our baby are most likely having our skin-to-skin connection moment, and the placenta might be the last thing we are thinking about.

Fourth stage

Some people do not consider this to be a stage, as the labor process has technically ended. However, there are essential tasks that need to be taken care of once the baby is out of the womb, still in the birthing room, for both mom and baby.

Mom care
Mom's postpartum care is ensuring the mother's well-being. It should focus on ours physical and emotional health as we begin recovery.

It typically includes tasks like monitoring for bleeding, checking for tears that might need stitching, and addressing any discomfort that may arise after giving birth. It is also possible to not have any tears and just need rest to recover our energy.

Baby care

The procedures may vary based on the mother's preferences, birth center or hospital polices, country of birth, etc., but will typically involve:

Apgar Score Assessment:
- The baby's overall health and well-being.
- The Apgar score evaluates their heart rate, breathing, muscle tone, reflexes, and skin color.

Initial Evaluation:
- The baby is checked for any immediate health concerns, and their weight, length, and head circumference are measured.

Eye Ointment:
- The application of *erythromycin* eye ointment to prevent eye infections.
- In the US, it is required by some state regulations.

Vitamin K Injection:
- Administration of a vitamin K injection to prevent bleeding disorders.

Hepatitis B Vaccine:
- Administering the first dose of the Hepatitis B vaccine.

Circumcision (if it's a boy):
- Parents have the option to circumcise their male baby.

Footprints and Identification:
- Footprints and identification bands are taken for record-keeping and security.

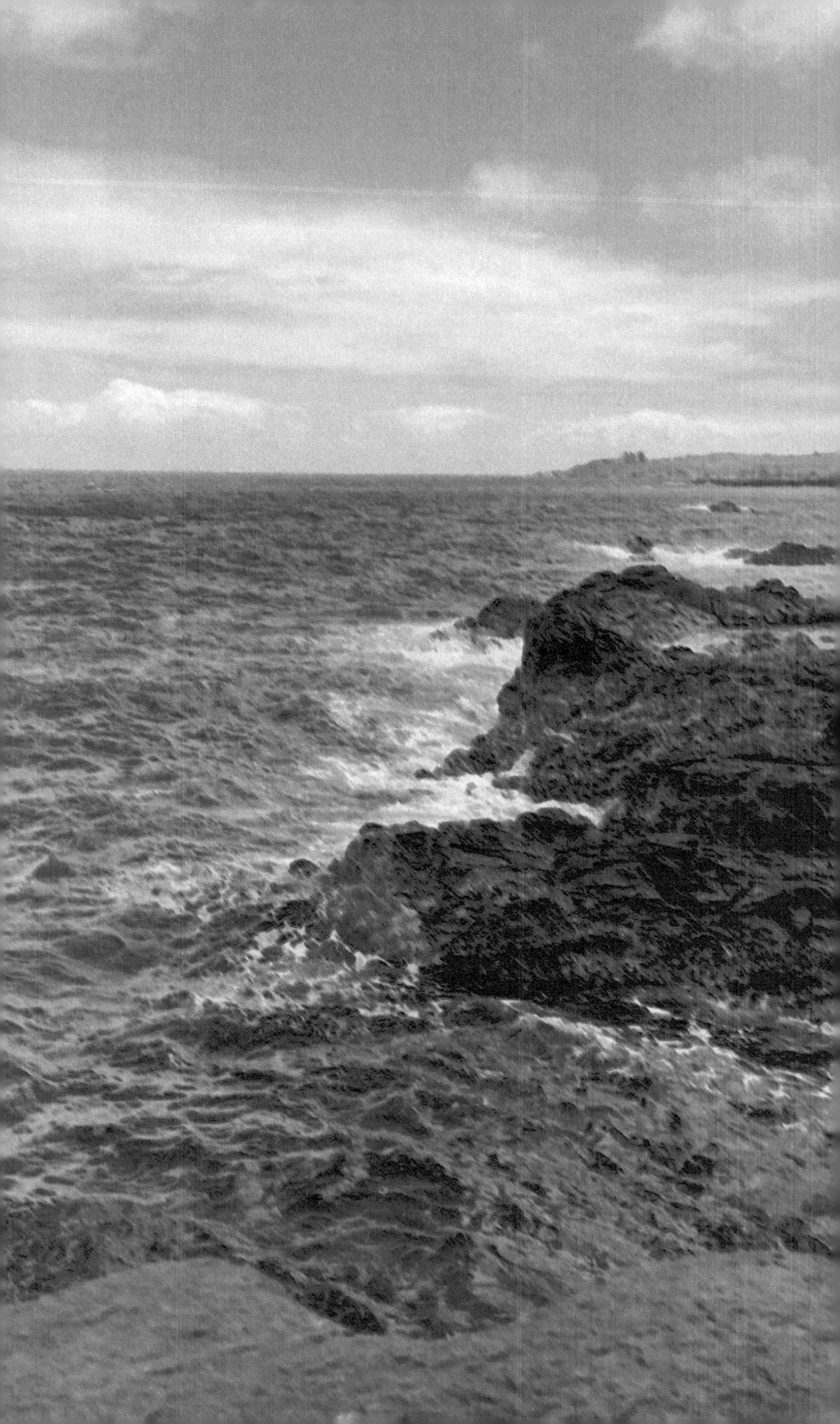

Contractions

*The power of redirecting our focus
and rewiring our brains*

It is important to recognize mom's mental health. There is a lot of talk about postpartum depression and how to deal with it after the fact, but what about treating the cause? A positive birth experience is of the utmost importance.

Many times, a negative birth experience is wrongly classified as an okay experience with the sentence, "Oh well, at least mom and baby are healthy." If we think about it, that actually sounds quite insensitive. A study found that 45% of new moms report their birth experience as traumatic. Our standards should be higher than just being okay with negative experiences that can lead to postpartum depression. The focus should be on a birth where mom and baby are both physically and *mentally* healthy.

A woman can give birth uninjured and unafraid. There are many studies that show us that having a positive birthing experience is often the result of checking off a list like this one:

- Getting informed.
- Having a sense of control.
- Meeting the expectations set during labor prep.
- Feeling empowered.
- Feeling confident.
- Feeling supported by partner(s) and medical team.

There is something "scary" about contractions. A lot of us struggle in advance with how much pain we will feel while going through the contractions (and delivery). Fortunately, there are techniques to help us. Aside from the techniques reviewed in previous chapters, a mighty tip is to stop thinking of it as painful and describe the sensations using different words. If we consistently use the word "pain" to label our feelings, we might reinforce the perception of discomfort and suffering. Instead, we should use alternative words to encourage more positive sensations. This will send different signals to our minds and bodies, promoting a more favorable experience. Setting our mind this way will help wire our brain to have more optimistic feelings and consequently a better birth.

> Some alternative words/sentences to use are:
> - It is on the uncomfortable side
> - It is pressuring
> - It is somewhat manageable
> - Needs work through it
> - It could be eased
> - Sensory awareness is at a 100%
> - I feel tightness
> - It feels somewhat sore

There are two distinct nervous systems: the Sympathetic Nervous System and the Parasympathetic Nervous System, which influence how our bodies respond during labor.

Sympathetic Nervous System (SNS)
- Governed by fear.
- Causes muscle tightness, especially in the cervix.
- Redirects blood to the extremities rather than where our body needs it most.
- Is responsible for immobilization and shutdown.

When fear accompanies contractions, it can make them stop. This is our body's way of protecting us. When we are in fear, we remain on high alert, making it challenging to continue with what frightens us. The Sympathetic Nervous System (SNS) triggers the release of adrenaline, which inhibits the production of endorphins. Without endorphins, contractions are less efficient, and we push without success. Consequently, our body stops producing oxytocin, the natural 'feel-good' hormone. Oxytocin is like a magical elixir that signals to our body, "this is okay." When fear prevents oxytocin production, we experience more pain. It is worth noting that doctors can administer synthetic oxytocin externally, known as Pitocin. Pitocin is often used to induce labor. However, while it does help initiate or enhance contractions, it comes at the cost of increased pain, unlike our natural oxytocin. This underscores the significance of activating the Parasympathetic Nervous System.

Parasympathetic Nervous System (PNS)
- Promotes smooth muscle relaxation.
- Supports adequate blood flow.
- Produces anti-stress enzymes such as acetylchloline, prolactin and oxytocin.
- Helps us feel connected and engaged.

The Sympathetic Nervous System (SNS) is activated during moments of stress or danger and can slow down our labor progress. On the contrary, the Parasympathetic Nervous System (PNS) will help us in moving the labor along with more ease.

To promote the activity of the Parasympathetic Nervous System during labor, we can, as already know and have practiced, engage in relaxation techniques, deep breathing, and positive visualization. Having a supportive and calming birthing environment, a compassionate birthing team, and a trusted partner can also encourage the activation of this nervous system (PNS).

To shift the balance towards the Parasympathetic Nervous System (PNS), it is essential to:
- Remain calm.
- Stay relaxed.
- Have an effective support team.
- Feel secure.

It all revolves around the same fundamental principle: ensuring a positive birthing experience by feeling good during the process. Ultimately, the pursuit of feeling good during childbirth is not just a personal preference; it can significantly impact the entire birthing journey, from the early stages of labor through to postpartum recovery.

Coping with contractions specifically
It's important to recognize that our initial response at the beginning of a contraction sets the tone for the entire contraction, including when it reaches its peak.

I. Am. Calm.

To ensure a more manageable experience, we will do our best to stay calm. We repeat to ourselves, "I am calm."
- We understand that getting tense when a contraction begins can escalate its intensity, subsequently increasing discomfort and pain. To counter this, we aim to start each contraction from a place of relaxation.
- We acknowledge that it might not always be easy to remain on the calmer side of the spectrum when a contraction starts, and that is okay.
- We accept this variability and approach each contraction as it comes, with a focus on staying relaxed during the resting period and working on our calmness levels for the next one.

Additionally, we'll enhance our ability to cope with contractions by practicing getting comfortable with the uncomfortable. To achieve this, we will engage in exercises such as the "comb trick" or the "ice trick", both explained in the *Coping with pain chapter.* This practice can be beneficial both in the lead-up to the birth and during the birthing process, helping us build resilience and adapt to sensations we may find challenging.

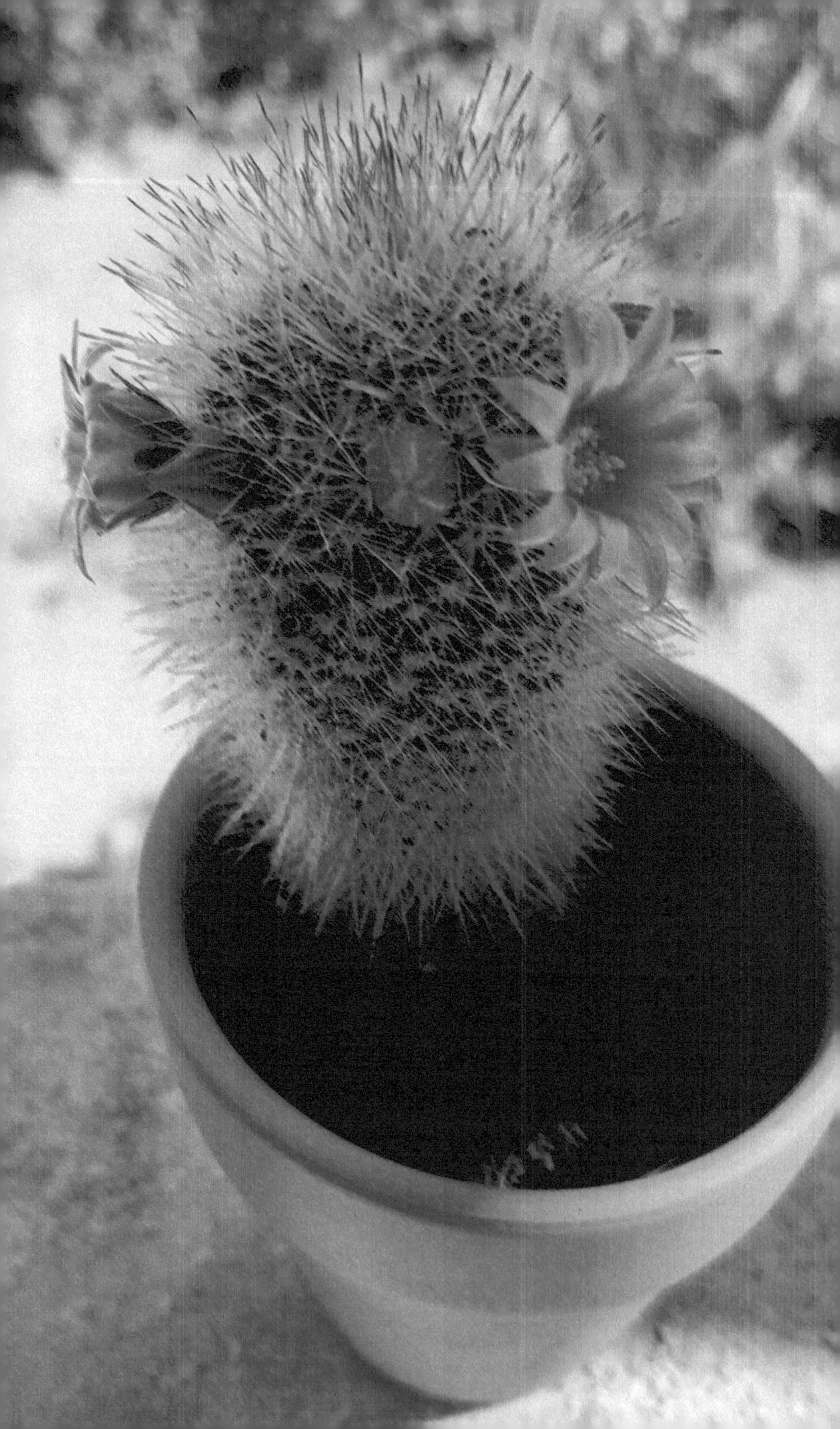

Coping With Pain

The power of meeting our bodies needs

Birth in real life has little to do with the painful picture Hollywood portrays it as in movies and shows. In fact, the more we learn about the birthing process the less believable those stories get.

Even though there are many sad and traumatic birth stories, there are many more wonderful and happy stories. Unfortunately, these amazing stories are not as known. As a general rule, our human brains are more capable of retaining negative stories. We must not let one negative story drown out ten positive ones. There are many books, blogs, and channels where positive birth experiences can be found.

Some people ask
"Why not use the advances in medicine
to make your life easier?"
We say
"Why not use what nature gave us as mighty women
to make our lives brighter?"

There are many ways to cope with pain, both natural and medicated. Knowing more about the different techniques available to us will put us in control during one of the most important moments of our lives. The best part about the natural options is that we can combine them as needed. We can start practicing these techniques as early as we want. Having our body prepared means an easier birth and a faster recovery. The techniques are:

- Support
- Rebozo
- Hydrotherapy
- Aromatherapy
- Music therapy
- Dim lights
- Focus and distraction
- TENS units
- Counter-pressure
- Massage
- Positioning
- Acupressure (the comb trick)
- The ice-trick
- Breathing techniques
- Affirmations

Support

Having a support person while in labor is extremely helpful. Some women just need the person to be there. They may prefer not to be touched or talked to but take comfort in knowing the person is there. Others prefer to this person to be more involved. A support person can contribute to creating a positive birth experience, and can guide us through breathing and relaxation techniques, especially if they have been helping us while practicing exercises during the pregnancy. They can also help us move into different positions to relieve some discomfort. They can also be part of other coping techniques like rebozo, counter-pressure, or massages.

The choice of a support person is a personal one, and it may include a partner, a *doula*, or a friend. What matters is the emotional and psychological support that comes from that trusted person.

Rebozo

The Rebozo is a shawl that can provide comfort and aid in the progress of labor. The assistance of our partner is crucial for this technique. To use the Rebozo, we fold the shawl lengthwise, place it across our belly, and pull it somewhat tightly. We can do this while in a standing position or on our hands and knees. The tightness of the Rebozo offers support and stability, helps relieve the weight from the heavy belly, and counteracts any discomfort that may occur due to the natural loosening of joints and ligaments in preparation for labor and birth.

Additionally, when squatting during labor, wrapping the Rebozo around our midsection can make squatting easier and conserve energy for the pushing stage.

Hydrotherapy

Hydrotherapy is a great way to relax the pregnant body and alleviate the uncomfortable aches that can arise during pregnancy, particularly by reducing pressure on the spine.

It's important to distinguish between hydrotherapy and a water birth. A water birth involves delivering the baby underwater, while hydrotherapy is used as a comfort measure during pregnancy and labor (not for delivery). Warm water during labor is known to provide comfort and support relaxation. Most experts recommend maintaining the water at around 100 degrees Fahrenheit (37.8 degrees Celsius) to prevent raising the body temperature to unsafe levels. If at any point we feel overheated, it is crucial to exit the water immediately.

Some hospitals and childbirth centers may offer baths, while others may have showers. It is advisable to have a partner present in the shower as bathroom floors can become slippery. Ensuring the safety of the pregnant woman is of utmost importance.

Essential oils help to resettle our minds so we can connect with our overjoyed body and soul. Here is a list of 10 *essential,* essential oils.

Bergamont
It brings light and sunshine to our environment. It portrays harmony and love to cherish our baby while reducing uncomfortable sensations.

Frankincense
This one is very helpful for the baby. It helps them to feel connected to the world they are going to be born into. Also, rubbing it on the lower back and abdomen can ease labor discomfort.

Lemon
It brings strength and gives us the energy to do things. Its fresh smell helps us get rid of the slothful pregnancy feeling, and it gets us moving.

Spearmint
It helps with morning sickness and keeps the environment happy and blissful.

Ginger
This oil contains many different positive qualities. It soothes, excites, energizes, and enhances anything we need.

Lavender
It brings peace to us, to the baby, and the people around us. It settles mom and baby and eases muscular tension. This is a soothing and relaxing oil that helps with aches.

Orange blossom
It brings joy and fun to the environment, and it brings

happiness to our spirit which releases endorphins.

Sweet Orange

It's mood-lifting and energy-boosting. It pours peace and joy over the environment. It also brings laughter and a happy feeling to mom.

Rose oil

It brings a sensation of love to us and the people we share our environment with. Also, massaging it into the lower back can help loosen muscles.

Neroli

It deflects negative habits and thoughts. It also helps us connect with our baby.

Jasmine

It evokes feelings of joy, happiness, peace, and self-confidence. It also can be used as a massage oil to reduce discomfort and ease back pressure.

Music therapy

Listening to music during labor has the power to change how we perceive pain. Music helps activate mental processes that make labor sensations more comfortable. Music activates the part of the brain associated with memory and emotion, stimulating the pituitary gland inside our brain to release endorphins and increase levels of serotonin. Listening to music during labor may also promote pain relief by helping us relax, reducing anxiety, and providing a positive source of distraction as we let ourselves flow with the different melodies and sounds.

We can prepare different playlists for our labor. This way, we have options that align with our mood depending on how we feel during different stages of the birthing process. It is also very important to get a device ready and a charger.

Playlists depending on the mood:
Energetic mood
- A list with hits that makes us move and dance, these songs are going to bring our energy up and remind us of moments of pure joy.

Nostalgic mood
- A list with calmer songs that have lyrics we connect to, songs that we can sing along in our head, softly, or out loud and that connect us to moments we cherish.

Relaxing mood
- A list of instrumental peaceful music that will help us relax and perhaps even get us in tune with our breathing.

Dim lights

The environment has big effects on the pathophysiology of birth. Dim lighting has a soothing impact on the birthing woman. A study out of Denmark showed that women who were in sensory birth rooms (with dim lights) were less likely to require a cesarean section, or an oxytocin infusion (pitocin) for augmentation than the ones in a standard delivery room.

Focus and distraction

Many methods of coping with pain rely on the laboring woman's ability to focus and use mind-diverting activities. It is common to release stress hormones during a life changing event like giving birth. These events can cause fear and anxiety. A good technique to ease stress is envisioning a pleasant scene, connecting to our uterus and visualizing the cervix opening, or visualizing the baby moving down.

Focus

Focusing empowers us to feel more in control of our birthing experience. Concentrating our on a focal point can promote a strong mind-body connection, allowing us to better manage and endure pain. Focusing one's attention is a deliberate activity and it is aided by verbal coaching, visualization, and self-hypnosis.

Distraction

Distraction is a more passive form of focusing attention. It happens when our attention is drawn away from our pain by something from the environment. An extensive list of happy anecdotes and jokes that make us laugh is a great source of positive endorphins. It not only helps defocus from the pain, but also builds a strong connection with our partner in this key moment in our lives.

TENS units

This is a battery-operated device. Transcutaneous Electrical Nerve Stimulation (TENS) units work by delivering small electrical impulses through electrodes that have adhesive pads to attach them to our skin. These electrical impulses flood the nervous system, reducing its ability to transmit pain signals. This device stimulates our body which encourages the production of endorphins (natural pain relievers).

Counter-pressure

Counter-pressure consists of steady, strong force applied to either one spot on the lower back, or on the side of each hip using both hands. This pressure helps alleviate back pain during labor. Applying counter-pressure during contractions can help balance the body and ease the pain.

Positioning

Changing positions is key. We know that listening to our body and adapting to what our body needs makes the most sense. Frequent position changes help baby descend and align in the pelvis, which tends to result in a shorter labor experience. (Remember the rocking technique exercise form the *Pregnancy Prep chapter* in the physical prep section). Movement releases endorphins and hormones which decrease the perception of pain and can even help with increasing the diameter of the pelvic outlet.

Rocking

We have practice rocking exercises during our pregnancy. Ideally, during labor, we would rock on a birth ball (or yoga ball), but we can also use a stool or a comfortable chair.
- We move back and forth
- We move side to side

We can adjust the rhythm to whatever feels better. We can also hold the position and breathe out as needed.

Squatting

Squatting is great to help with birth progress as gravity helps our baby move down the birth canal. However, it can be challenging to maintain correct posture, or to keep the position for a prolonged period of time without losing balance, especially while contractions are happening. It is great to be able to practice on our own, but it is very helpful to have our partner's assistance while in labor. Some help options are:

- With a partner, using rebozo
- With a partner, using a chair
- Using a squatting bar

With a partner, using rebozo

We place the rebozo around our back. Our partner, who is in front of us, facing us, takes the two ends of the rebozo. They tense the rebozo and we squat down. This gives us support and helps us keep our balance.

With a partner, using a chair

With our partner sitting on a chair, we squad in front of the chair, giving our back to our partner who is supporting us by putting their arms around ours and holding us back. This exercise might allow us to squat a little deeper.

Squat bar

This bar is typically placed at the end of the hospital bed. We can use the bar for multiple positions. We can put our feet at the end of the bed and hold onto the squat bar with just our hands, or we can place our entire upper body on the top part of the bar (like we would do on an actual bar, or a counter-top). We can also have our feet on the floor while holding the top part of the bar and hang from there.

Lying on our side

The side-lying position is especially useful in promoting rest and relaxation between pushing during contractions. We rest most likely on our left side with our body slightly curled, or in the "fetal" position. For side-lying, we can do it by ourselves or we can use our partner's support by having them hold one of our legs up. We can also use a peanut ball, and some hospital beds might have a foot rest where we can place our feet.

This is very beneficial for our baby too, as it removes pressure from the uterus, kidneys, or other internal organs that can compress the umbilical cord.

Birthing stool

A birthing stool, also called a birthing chair, is something in between a normal stool and a toilet. It helps us push in a very familiar position. Ideally, our partner is behind us so that, in between contractions, we can lean back to rest with their support. We are comfortably sitting upright, which increases the effectiveness of uterine contractions. Also, the low height of the stool flexes our legs and expands the size of our pelvis. This, along with gravity promoting the downward movement of our baby, will assist in shortening labor.

Birthing stools typically feature a cutout portion of the seat to allow attending midwives or physicians to catch the baby from under the parent easily.

Alternating walking and standing

Walking keeps us upright, allowing our body to work *with* gravity to move baby down and out. It can help ease the intensity of labor as well as keep labor progressing by moving our pelvic bones with one of our most familiar moves: walking. After all, we have been walking on an everyday basis since forever.

Walking can even help to get labor started. Many woman *curb-walk* for this very reason. This is walking right on the edge of a curb, one leg on the upper side and one on the lower side. While in early labor, walking may help push labor along a bit quicker into active labor. We will probably need to stop walking during a contraction. When in active labor, walking can become challenging, but we still can take short walks and just stand during contractions, holding on to our partner, or something nearby like a wall for support.

On hands and knees

This position can be done on a yoga mat for practice, and on a bed for labor. Typically, on a hospital bed, we would face the back of the bed, having the backrest angled up. With our knees on the bed, we place our hands and elbows on the highest part of the bed.

This position can be helpful if there are decelerations in the fetal heart rate, and it may also help to turn our baby into a better position for descent.

While we are in our hands and knees, we can also exercise in different ways:
- Rocking technique
- Wiggle the tail technique
- Cat/cow movements technique
- Frog movements technique

Detailed exercises and physical prep in the *Pregnancy Prep Chapter.*

Hypnobirthing

Relaxation and self-hypnosis techniques help relax the body before, during, and after labor. The goal is to get our body and mind fully relaxed to help birth progress faster. We can painlessly allow our body and mind to be connected so our body doesn't fight the natural process.

This technique combines others explained throughout the chapter.
- Controlled breathing to help trigger our parasympathetic nervous system, which will give us

a calm sensation.
- The use of affirmations, and positive thoughts.
- Visualization to overpower the pain and stress hormones.

Vocalization

It consists of low, deep moans or groans. Low moaning sounds help cope with pain and progress labor. By staying away from high-pitched yelling, squealing or screaming, we allow the connection between our mind and body be more effective. This can help in relaxing the pelvic floor and perineum area, and ultimately help to avoid tears.

Sometimes, if we experience pain, our pitch can get higher (which tenses our muscles). It might be helpful if our support person makes eye contact with us and guides us toward making low tones.

For this technique, we will take a breath in and, as we exhale, make different sounds:
- Inhale, exhale making an "H" or "Haa..." sound
- Inhale, exhale making an "U" or "Uh..." sound
- Inhale, exhale making an "M" or "Mmm..." sound
- Inhale, exhale making an "A" or "Ahh..." sound
- Inhale, exhale making an "O" or "Oh..." sound

The "comb-trick" technique

This "trick" is actually acupressure. Acupressure is the technique of applying pressure on specific points on the body to treat health problems naturally and restore the flow of energy.

Any comb can do the job, but one with thicker, less sharp teeth, and possibly made out of wood would reduce possible tenderness caused by the comb when used for longer periods of time. We hold a comb in our hand with the teeth placed at the top of our palm, right below the edge between our fingers and our palm.

This is a useful technique for active labor, when our contractions are strong enough that we can't talk through them. The comb creates a distraction that takes the focus away from the contraction.

The "ice-trick" technique

This "ice-trick" consists inholding an ice cube in our hand for increasing durations, adding 15 seconds with each interval while taking 15-second breaks in between. This trick is explained in more detail in the *Breathing Techniques Chapter.*

Breathing techniques

Giving concentration to our breathing has incredible benefits in coping with pain, especially during contractions. Detailed breathing methods in the *Breathing Techniques Chapter.*

Affirmations

Affirmations are short sentences with a powerful and strong message that speak to us and help us get into a positive mindset. Extended list of affirmations in the *Affirmations Chapter.*

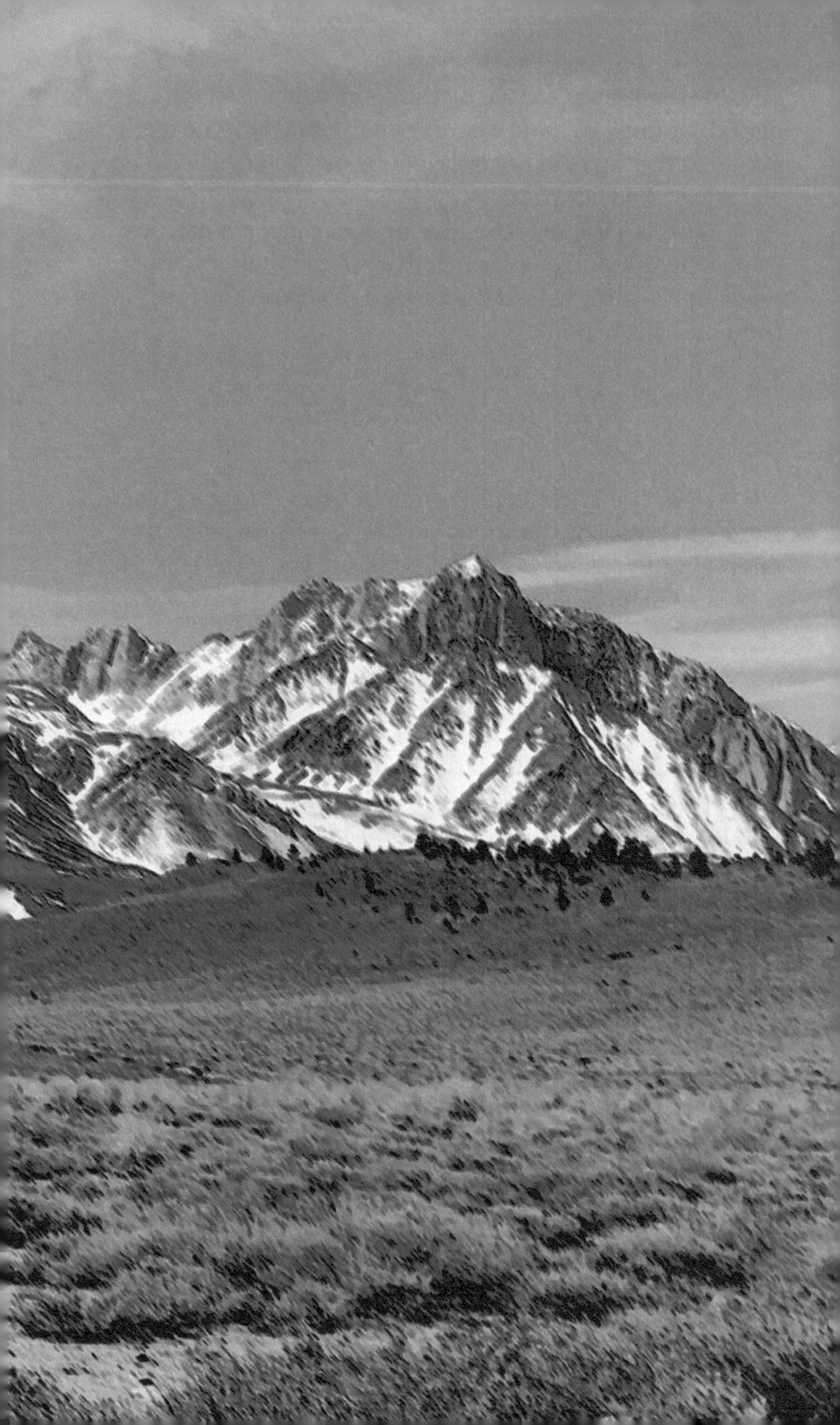

Breathing Techniques

The power of staying calm and relaxed

Breathing brings oxygen to the muscles. When we have contractions, our uterus—which is a muscle—is contracting. When a muscle contracts, it tightens and restricts food and oxygen, is this lack of oxygen what causes pain. By focusing on breathing, we are providing the oxygen back to the muscle. Deep and slow breathing distracts, relaxes, and makes contractions more effective.

Muscle relaxation in between contractions

As the contraction finishes, we use visualization to imagine the contraction physically leaving our body. We visualize it dissipating and fading away.

Now that the contraction has passed, we take advantage of the resting period to relax each muscle from our forehead down to our toes. Our partner's assistance is particularly helpful with this technique. They can guide us through the process of relaxing each muscle, allowing us to focus on the relaxation itself without worrying about missing any muscle group. At the same time, if during one of the rest periods we overlook a muscle group or we do not have the time to go through some of the groups because a contraction is approaching, that is completely fine. The primary goal is to stay relaxed, so it is okay to prioritize what feels manageable in the moment. Each rest period is a new opportunity to focus on relaxation, and there is no need to stress if we cannot cover every muscle group every time. We will take each contraction as it comes and adapt.

That said, having a list of muscle groups can serve as a helpful guide.

- Forehead
- Eyebrows
- Yaw
- Neck
- Shoulders
- Hands (wrists and fingers)
- Hips
- Legs
- Feet (ankles and toes)

Diaphragmatic breathing

Diaphragmatic breathing also known as deep or abdominal breathing is a technique where the stomach, rather than the chest, moves with each breath, it expands while inhaling and contracts while exhaling. Using the diaphragm allows for a more efficient inhalation and exhalation. Focusing on breathing while going though a contraction helps us putting the attention on getting calm and away from the pressuring sensation. To allow our breathing to help even more, we are going help our uterus by breathing with our diaphragm. When we exhale we are going to send our air down, not forward, and expand the sides of our belly.

To feel the air as we are breathing, we place a hand in front of our mouth. We are going to inhale, then on the exhale we will let the air go right straight to our hand. This way, we will feel all of our air and strength focusing on exiting through our mouth.

Now, we are going to make air work more effectively.
- We place a hand in front of our mouth again.
- We inhale and , on the exhale, focus on pushing the air downward and we are going to do an "aaa" or "mmm" sound to help us accomplish this.
- Very little air to none is getting to the hand in front of our mouth because the air is going down.
- This is a very powerful technique that not only keeps us calm but also helps our uterus push down our baby.

The "ice-trick" technique

For this technique, we will keep our breathing at a steady pace. The amount of seconds to inhale or exhale does not matter, as long as we keep the same rhythm. The key point is to be able to hold some ice in our hands. The longer we hold the ice in our hands, the easier it is to start breathing more quickly or unevenly, we need to try to avoid that from happening.

The technique consists on placing some ice in our hand for short periods of time, elongating the periods every time.

Hold the ice for 15 seconds
Rest for 15 seconds

Then hold the ice for 30 seconds
Rest for 15 seconds

Then 45 seconds
Rest for 15 seconds

Then 60 seconds
Discard the ice

Focused respiration

When we focus on our respiration during childbirth, we practice a mindfulness technique. This technique involves concentrating our attention on our breath to help manage discomfort, anxiety, or any challenging feelings that may arise during labor. By doing so, we aim to keep our minds centered and calm.

> If there is something I know how to do is breathing, I've been doing that all my life, so let's just do that.
> Let's just breathe!

We are going to try another way with a more focused respiration in relation to the contractions. Contractions will generally last for about 45 seconds to 1 minute. We are going to follow a 1:2 ratio in the following way:

1st breathing
4 seconds inhale
8 seconds exhale

2nd breathing
4 seconds inhale
8 seconds exhale

3rd breathing
4 seconds inhale
8 seconds exhale

4th breathing
4 seconds inhale
8 seconds exhale

Pushing stage breathing

Many doctors and nurses in hospitals encourage this type of breathing for the expulsion phase of labor, especially if the mom-to-be is laying on a bed. This technique is used once the cervix is fully dilated, marking the beginning of the second stage of labor.

Firstly, we will start with an organizing breath—a big sigh as soon as the contraction begins, letting go of all tension and going limp from head to toe as we exhale. If we put this technique in practice, we can combine it with visualization and focus on positive imaginary like our baby moving downward.

Then, we will breathe slowly, following the rhythm of the contraction and modify the pace or lightness of our breath for comfort.

When the irresistible urge to push arises, we will take a big breath, tuck our chin to our chest, curl our body, lean forward, and bear down. We will hold our breath or release air slowly with grunting or moaning. Grunting may result in our bodies feeling contracted, and our vocal cords may experience tightness. It is crucial, when using this approach, to relax ourselves as much as possible and maximize the relaxation of our pelvic floor to assist our baby's descent and ease tension in the perineum.

Square breathing technique

We are going to alternate the ice exercises with breathing that doesn't involve freezing our hand.

We are going to mentally draw a square while we do our breathing. To do this, We are going to look around and find a rectangular form to use as our guide. A cabinet or a picture is great. Once we have identified what we will use as our guide.

We are going to focus all our attention on that shape and follow the outline of it as we breathe.

4 seconds: Inhale, mentally draw the first line of the square from the bottom up.

4 seconds: Hold the breath at the corner.

8 seconds: Exhale through the mouth, mentally draw the second line. From the left to the right.

4 seconds: Inhale, mentally draw the next line from the top to the bottom.

4 seconds: Hold the breath at the corner.

8 seconds: Exhale through the mouth, mentally draw the last line and close the square.

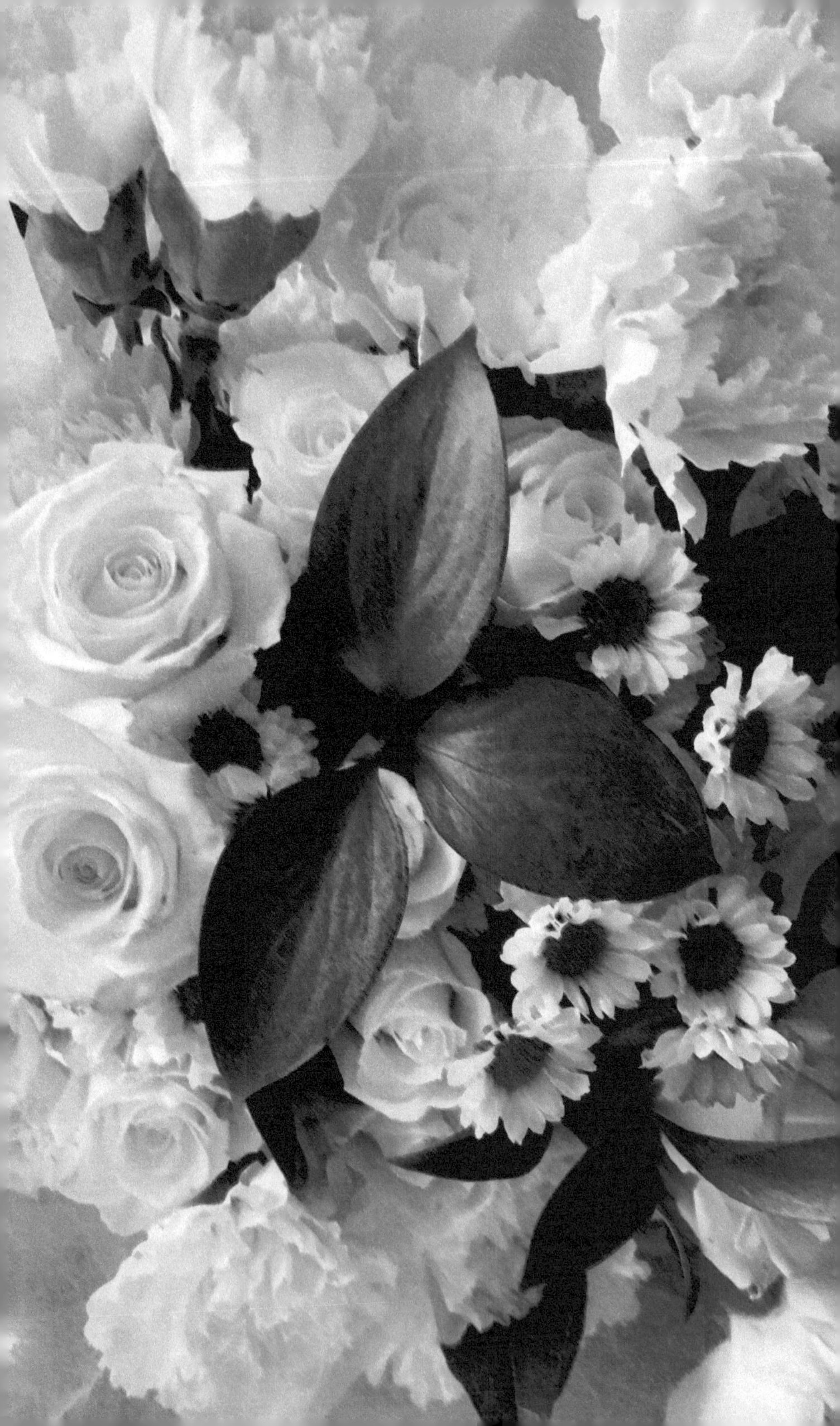

Affirmations

The power of repeating positive and assertive sentences

Preparing for birth can be an exciting yet nerve-wracking experience for many expectant mothers. With so many unknowns and changes happening to the body and mind, it is common to feel anxious or overwhelmed. When these sensations appear we need to remember that there is a lot of beauty to be found in the unknown.

One tool that can be helpful in managing these emotions and preparing for a positive birth experience is the practice of affirmations.

> Affirmations work because they help reprogram our thoughts, ourselves and the birth process.

Affirmations bring us peace and calm. By incorporating affirmations into our daily routine, foster a positive mindset, boost our self-assurance, and prepare ourselves mentally and emotionally for the arrival of our child.

It is important to accept that we will know some of them by heart as we repeat them over and over again while others might not stick. It is also possible that we might not be able to recite affirmations we knew by heart while we are in labor. This is perfectly normal.

Throughout labor, our body experiences a blend of intense and relaxed movements. Our mind may also be filled with thoughts, and our objective is to maintain, not diminish, our sense of calm. We know our thoughts control our actions and feelings so it is key to stay and maintain positivity.

> True change happens
> when we shift our thoughts
> by using positive affirmations.

We will seek assistance when necessary, and a part of seeking help involves asking our support person to read the affirmations to us. This process is important to us and it is important for our labor progress. We will recite the affirmations as we see fit, regardless of who is in the room. Maybe we are happy to just repeat the affirmations in our mind—just to ourselves or to ourselves and the baby.

Affirmations List

I am prepared for this moment,
this is my moment

I am committed to welcome this baby,
my baby

I will allow my body to do
what it well knows how to do

I have been working to get ready
for this moment

I am delighted I can put
all my preparation to work

I have the courage to engage
with the labor process

Each contraction brings me closer
to meeting my baby

I am at peace with my body
and my mind

I accept the natural process of birth
and I will stand strong by my natural
birth plan

My body is wise,
and knows what to do

My body knows how to give birth,
and I trust it completely

I am strong and I am a good mother

I am strong and I can do this

I fully appreciate each movement my
body makes because it brings my baby
closer to me

I will provide my baby a safe space to
enter this world

My baby is ready and I will help him/
her to meet me on the outside of the
womb

My body, my baby, my choice

I am at peace with my environment

The doctors and nurses are there to
help and guide me if I require it

I know my body and I can make
my own decisions

I feel empowered, and I know that I am
the one who is bringing my baby into
the world

I open my heart to love the labor
process

I connect to the rhythm of my
contractions

The rhythm of the contractions are my
dance today and I enjoy it

I open my heart to connect the rhythm
of my soul with my baby's heartbeat

I am building a huge entrance for my
little one

I am relaxed, my body is relaxed, my
baby is relaxed

I feel the love and support of my
partner, and my birth team

This is my perfect birth and it's
happening at the perfect time

My breathing is a powerful tool and I
embrace its power

I breathe in strength
and I breathe out confidence

I am safe
my baby is safe

I invite softness into my physical body

I surrender to the experience of labor
and trust the process

We visualize our baby moving down
and out of our body with ease and
grace

My breathing is my anchor, and it
helps me stay calm and focused

My body is made for this,
and I am doing an incredible job

I am surrounded by positive energy,
and I welcome it into my birth space

I am a warrior, and I am meeting each
moment of labor with courage and
strength

I am here in the now and emotionally
minded with my loves ones

My body is strong and capable of
giving birth to my baby

I am proud of myself

I trust my instincts and my ability to
make the right decisions for myself
and my baby

I am surrounded by love and support
as I prepare for the birth of my child

My baby and I have been growing
stronger and healthier and we are
ready for this moment

I am calm and relaxed

The more relaxed I am, the better
experience my baby will have

I am able to thrive
through the labor process

I embrace the changes in my body

I welcome each contraction
because it gets me closer to my baby

My baby will be born
at exactly the right time
and in exactly the right way
for us

I can naturally give birth to my baby

I trust that my body knows
how to give birth

I have all I need to give birth
to my baby

I embrace my ability to give birth

I have the power to accomplish
everything I need

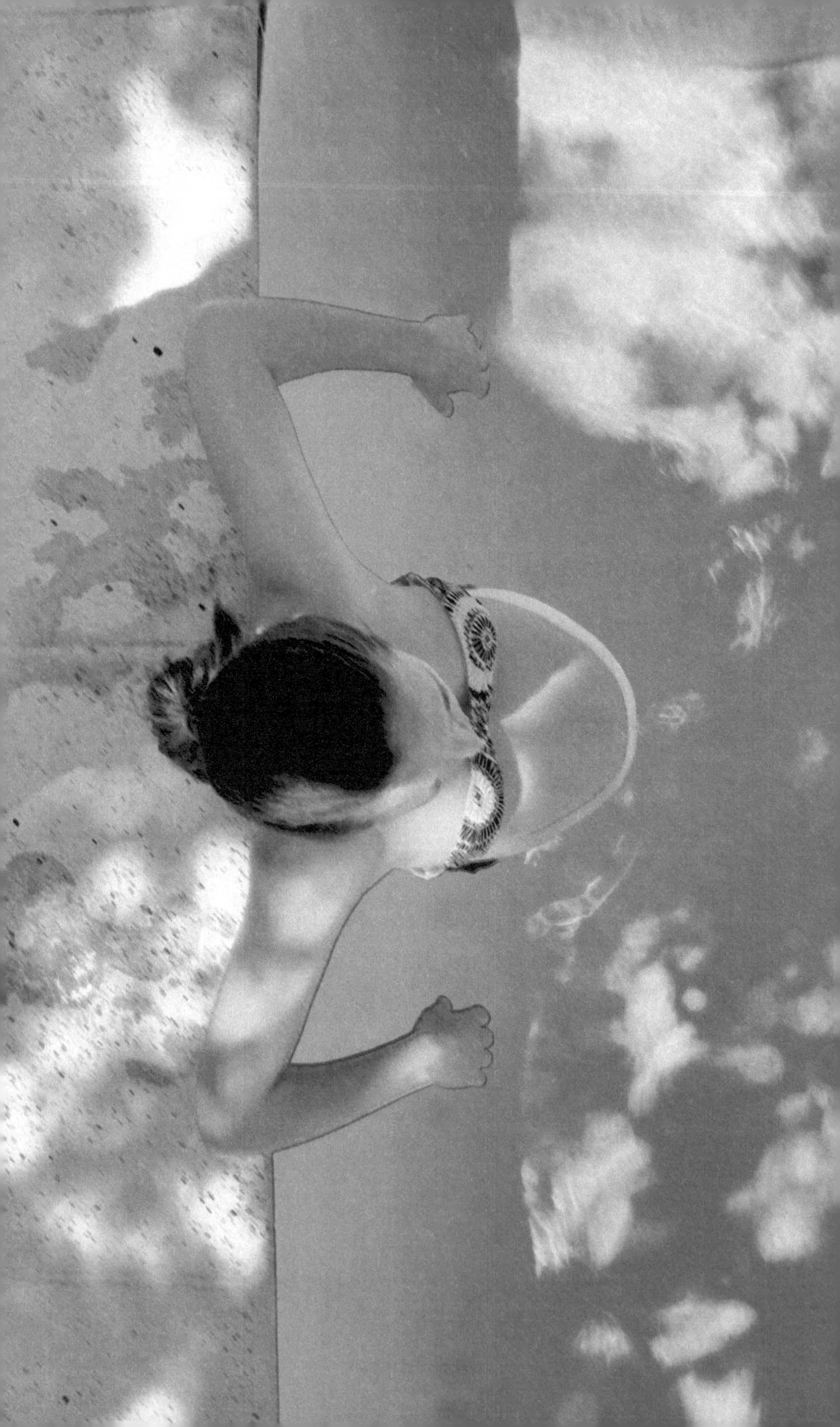

Birth Plan and Options

The power of being ready and knowing what we want

Throughout our pregnancy, we have been preparing for a natural, unmedicated birth. We understand that, if there are severe complications that put our baby or us at risk, the doctors will let us know that they need to perform an intervention, and we will listen to their expertise. However, we will also advocate for ourselves and ask questions, so that we fully understand if a medical intervention is needed.

Weighing Options

Before our labor day, we will make a birth plan that clearly indicates our birth preferences. We will talk to our birth partner about it and we will make sure they understand it so they can advocate for our preferences if any questions arise while we are focused on relaxing and progressing through the stages of labor. We will make three copies of our birth plan. When we arrive to the hospital, one copy will be for the practitioner or nurse, another one for our partner and another one for ourselves.

Our birth plan indicates that we don't want medical offerings and that we will be the ones asking for medication to cope with pain if we need it.

If a practitioner comes to tell us they need to intervene, we will ask two questions:
- Am I ok?
- Is my baby ok?

We know sometimes doctors want to get things moving, prioritizing their biases and preferences instead of the preferences that work for us and our body.

The following questions we will ask are:
- Is this medically necessary? If so, why?
- What other options do I have?
- How long do I have to make a decision?
- What happens if I decide not to proceed?

If we feel we are not being listened to and we are just another name on a list, we will follow up with another question:
- What medications or procedures do you feel would be best for me given my health and pregnancy specifically?

We will weigh the benefits and risks of each option. We understand that there are many methods for the birthing process and we will choose the option that best aligns with our birth goals and safety.

Being inform is one of our greater powers. We are allowed to have our own preferences for our birth. We should be supported in our informed choices. If during this very important event in our life, our body feels right, our labor will progress better and faster.

We know there are different points of view about birth. Some people prefer to have an epidural, some others prefer to give birth unmedicated. Epidurals have become the most common method, but we would rather feel the experience. We want to bring our baby into this world as naturally as possible and it is worth the discomfort.

Birthing is a powerful experience. Having a birth plan not only helps us ensure we know our options but also empowers us to understand what the different options are and to choose the best one for ourselves.

Preparing our birth plan

The heather
It should identify:
Who the birth plan is for (ourselves)
- Our medical record number
- Who is going to be in the delivery room (partner)
- Our partners contact phone number
- Baby's name
- Baby's gender
- EDD (Estimated Due Date)

Most important preferences
It should state the most important preferences. Each mother will have her own. For example:
- Natural birth (vaginal unmedicated birth)
- No medication offerings

- Freedom of movement
- Natural water rupture
- No episiotomy
- Skin-to-skin

1st stage: labor
This can be divided in a few sections:
- Interventions
  - None/Ask if emergency
  - IV Fluids
  - Antibiotics
  - Pitocin
  - Episiotomy
  - Blood transfusion
  - Membrane sweep
  - AROM
  - Prostaglandis
  - Foley bulb/Cook catheter
  - Hep-lock
  - Forceps
  - Vacuum

- Fetal monitoring
  - None
  - Being able to move
  - Internal
  - Handheld doppler
  - Intermittent
  - Continuous

- Cervical exams
  - None
  - Limited
  - As needed

- Birth environment
  - Music

- Dim lights
  - Diffusers/Oils
  - Quiet voices
  - Limited people in the room
  - Home or hospital clothing

- Nutrition
  - Drinking
  - Eating
  - Ice chips/clear foods
  - IV fluids

- Relaxation techniques
  - Hypnobirthing
  - Vocalization
  - Focus breathing
  - Visualization
  - Massage/Comfort touch
  - Hydrotherapy
  - Physical movement

- Pain management
  - Medications only offer is asked
  - Counter-pressure
  - Hot/Cold packs
  - Meditation/Physical exercises/Stretches
  - Nitrous Oxide
  - Sterile water injections
  - IV pain medication
  - Epidural

2nd stage: pushing and delivery

This can also be divided in a few sections:
- Labor and birth positions
  - Squatting
  - Lying on our side
  - Birthing stool

- Alternating walking and standing
- Lunging
- Forward leaning
- On hands and knees
- Laying on our back

- Pushing
  - Spontaneous pushing
  - Laboring down
  - Directed pushing

- Perineal care
  - Episiotomy/Prefer tear
  - Massage
  - Warm compresses

3rd stage: after baby delivery and delivery of the placenta

These can also be divided in a few sections:
- After delivery of the baby
  - Catching the baby (mom, dad, doctor)
  - Cutting the umbilical cord (dad, doctor)
  - Delayed cord clamping
  - Cord blood donation
  - Cord blood saving for private banking

- Delivery of the placenta
  - Saving the placenta
  - Lotus Birth

4th stage: mom and baby care
- These can also be divided in a few sections:
  - Baby
  - Skin-to-skin contact
  - breastfeeding asap
  - Leave vernix on baby/Delay bath
  - Circumcision (if it is a boy)

- Erythromycin eye cream
- Vitamin K
- Hepatitis B vaccine

Mom's care may also involve stitches or other types of care to ensure mom's body is well after the delivery of the baby and placenta. This is typically determined on a case-by-case basis by the doctor or midwife.

Understanding the meaning

To make inform decisions, we need to know what "stuff" is. Here are the choices we have for our birth plan with their definitions.

Interventions (1st stage)

None/Ask if emergency
We can choose to inform the personal we do not plan on having any interventions unless medical necessary.

IV Fluids
Helps keep me hydrated and allows for easier administration of antibiotics. Recommended for faster access in case of an emergency. Detachable intravenous (IV) for mobility. Optional if we prefer our water and plan on no medications. May be recommended to have it ready but not connected for emergency purposes.

Antibiotics
Medicaments that can be administered through the IV. We will be told specific antibiotics are mandatory if during our 3rd trimester, we tested positive for B-Strep to protect our baby. B-Strep is a bacteria that lives in women, this is not really a concern other than when giving birth vaginally.

Pitocin

Artificial oxytocin. It is used to induce labor. Many women report pitocin as the cause of painful labor. It assist in generating contractions and it can help move labor along, however, since it is not natural oxytocin, the contractions would be more hurtful.

Episiotomy

A cut in the perineum area performed to avoid tears. We might prefer to forgo an episiotomy and risk tearing instead. If we have been doing our perineum massages, it is in our favor to experience little to no tearing. This procedure is not a default in many hospitals anymore.

Blood transfusion

Receiving blood through an intravenous (IV) line into one of your blood vessels.

Membrane sweep

When the healthcare provider inserts a gloved finger into the cervix to loosen the amniotic sac from the uterus. It is used to induce labor when the cervix has started to dilate but contractions have not yet begun.

AROM (Artificial Rupture Of the Membranes)

When a nurse manually breaks our water by puncturing the amniotic sac with a hook. It is used to speed up labor.

Prostaglandis

A group of lipids with hormone-like actions. They play several essential roles in regulating bodily processes. This is used to speed up labor by increasing uterine hyper-stimulation.

Foley bulb

A device that helps dilate the cervix, used to induce labor. It consists of a catheter (a skinny tube) with a small, uninflated balloon at the end. The catheter, filled with a saline solution, is inserted into the cervix. Then the balloon inflates which opens the cerise (due to the pressure applied to it).

Cook catheter
A device that helps dilate the cervix, used to induce labor. It is similar to a Foley bulb, but this one uses two balloons, one on either side of the cervical opening.

Hep lock (heparin lock)
A place holder for an IV, in case an IV is needed later. It is a compromise, where we do not need to be hock up on to an IV, but in case of emergency, the nurses can quickly access it. It is an IV catheter that has a heparin solution when the IV is not in use. Heparin is a blood thinner medication that helps to prevent blood clots but it can cause excessive bleeding. Heparin locks are not used in peripheral IVs because the risk of bleeding.

Forceps
A form of assisted delivery. Obstetrical forceps are long, curved devices used to grasp the baby from inside the birth canal and help guide baby out.

Vacuum
A form of assisted delivery. It is a plastic cup placed on top of the baby's head that applies suction and traction to help pull the baby out while mom pushes. If needed, and used successfully, it might avoid a c-section.

Fetal monitoring (1st stage)
Being able to move
The ability to choose an option that would allow us to keep moving and changing positions.

Internal Monitoring
Continuous monitoring of fluctuations of the fetal heart

rate (FHR) in relation to our contractions, might be necessary if suspecting fetal distress. We may experience slight discomfort when the electrode is placed on our uterus. There is a small risk of infection or bruising to the baby.

Handheld doppler
External fetal monitor that is placed against our belly to listen to baby's heartbeat.

Intermittent
Only have fetal monitoring as needed. This can be done by the used of a Doppler (explained above).

Continuous
Having fetal monitoring continuously thought the labor. This normally means we are not able to move around.

Cervical Exams (1st stage)
A cervical exam is when the nurse, doctor, or midwife measures cervix dilation and effacement. It is done by introducing a gloved hand inside the cervix and it is measure by feeling how many fingers fit inside the cervix. The cervix must be 100% effaced and 10 centimeters dilated before a vaginal delivery.

Cervical effacement: During pregnancy, the cervix is typically long and firm. As labor approaches, the cervix undergoes effacement, becoming softer, shorter, and thinner. Effacement is often expressed as a percentage, with 0% indicating no effacement, and 100% indicating complete effacement.

Limited
Cervical exams can increased the risk of infection by putting a hand in the vagina. They can also cause discomfort and disruption to the labor progress and frustration if progress is slow. Limiting the cervical exams can help alleviate this pressure.

As needed

Normally done every 2-3h to check progress. It is important to remember that too many cervical exams can increase the risk for an infection.

Birth environment (1st stage)

Music

Playing music that helps us get into a mood conducive to progressing through labor.

Dim lights

Avoiding having bright lights to create a relaxing atmosphere.

Diffusers/Oils

Utilizing aromatherapy and taking advantages of the properties of the oils.

Quiet voices

Reducing loud voices and noises to avoid unnecessary distractions.

Limited people in the room

To avoid any uncomfortable feelings by having man people in the birth thing room. It is common for hospital births to have a lot of people in the room at the moment of birth.

Home or hospital clothing

Using the clothing that makes me feel the most comfortable.

Nutrition (1st stage)

Labor is hard work. To stay strong and be effective we need liquid and calories. We might feel nauseous, or have no appetite. However, a light, easy to digest snack during early labor can go a long way. Being able to eat or drink during labor can reduce labor time, avoid the need of Pitocin to accelerate the process, and can even benefit the baby. Studies shows non-fasting moms have babies with higher Apgar scores.

Apgar: A scoring system that measures the baby's health. This evaluation is done to the baby at one minute of life, and then again at five minutes of life.

Drinking
Being able to drink by ourselves while in labor, instead of getting liquids through an IV. The ACOG (The American College of Obstetricians and Gynecologist) guidelines allow liquids and light solids during labor.

Eating
Being able to eat while in labor. Eating can be very productive as it can help labor advance. However, it can also be contra producing in the rare case of needing general anesthesia for an emergency procedure (this is a 7 in 10 million birth situation).

Ice chips/clear foods
Having ice chips in the mouth can be a relaxing and distracting method to cope with pain during labor.

IV fluids
Being administered liquids and nutrients through an IV.

Relaxation techniques (1st stage)
Summarized, extended explanation in *Coping With Pain* chapter.

Hypnobirthing
Relaxation and self-hypnosis techniques to help relax the body before and during labor and birth.

Vocalization
This is a natural way to self-soothe by using low-pitch sounds to relax the body and possibly avoid extensive perineal tears.

Focus breathing

Deep and slow breathing distracts, relaxes, and makes contractions more effective.

Visualization

Using the mind to create positive imaginary and thoughts that encourage our body to produce endorphins and serotonin, which modulates our mood and takes pain away.

Massage/Comfort touch

A massage or light, caring contact to relieve tension.

Hydrotherapy

A warm bath or shower can help easing contraction discomfort. It provides ache relief and relaxation.

Physical movement and walking

Changing positions approximately every 30 minutes can assist with discomfort and aid in labor progression. Additionally, altering positions, standing, and walking whenever something doesn't feel good can help make it feel better.

Pain management (1st stage)
Medications only offer is asked

If we are aiming for a natural birth as much as possible, we will communicate in our birth plan to only get offered medications if we ask for them. In a hospital setting, the staff is accustomed to administering medications routinely, and we may need to remind them not to do so.

Counter-pressure

It is when our partner applies steady pressure on our lower back or the sides of our hips during a contraction. To be effective, they must push hard. Counter-pressure is a great tool to relieve muscle tension, open our hips a bit more to let baby down, and relieve back tightness.

Hot/Cold packs

The use of a warm towel or a hot/cold pack to help relax tense or painful areas.

Physical movements

The use physical techniques to ease the labor process.

Nitrous Oxide

An already established method in Europe, lately getting more common in the United States. It is an odorless gas given via a face-mask during labor. The mom is in control of the mask and would place it over the mouth and nose only when needed. Once removed, after a few exhales the gas would leave the mom's system. The effect of nitrous oxide is not to take contraction pain away but rather to make us care less about them. If considering this option, narcotic pain medication cannot be given simultaneously, pain medication has to worn off before using nitrous oxide.

Sterile water injections

It is a natural, safe treatment to alleviate back trouble. It can be performed quickly, without high risk to our baby or us. When administered, it might burn or tingle. Sterile water is injected under the skin in the lumbar area of our back.

IV pain medication

Different facilities use different medications through the IV, with Fentanyl being a commonly used one. Fentanyl is a short-acting opioid narcotic, stronger than morphine. The short duration of the medication is crucial during labor to prevent strong narcotics from crossing the placenta and impacting the baby. While this medication can relax us during contractions, it may also cause drowsiness, sleepiness, or dizziness. If it crosses the placenta, it can make the baby drowsy and sleepy as well. If using this type of medication, our baby would need to be on a fetal monitor to observe baby's heart rate.

Epidural

It is a type of anesthesia administered through a
needle inserted right below the spinal cord. This procedure is
typically performed by an anesthesiologist or nurse anesthetist
and takes about 15 minutes. Prior to receiving an epidural,
it is necessary to be connected to an intravenous (IV) line
to receive fluids and additional medications that enable the
epidurals' administration.

Epidurals provide regional anesthesia, numbing
sensations in the uterus, abdomen, and lower back. They
can also lead to a weakening of the legs. Additionally, having
an epidural often requires the placement of a catheter for
urination, which may limit the range of pushing positions to
those suitable for being in bed, such as lying on the back or on
one's side.

While some women may still experience pressure from
contractions and sensations in the pelvic floor, for others, the
epidural may not work or only work on one side of the body.
It is important to be aware of potential risks associated with
epidurals, including the possibility of spinal headaches, nerve
injuries, and weakness in the body.

Labor and birth positions (2nd stage)
Squatting

Being in a squat position, normally using a squat bar
attach to the end of the hospital bed, or supported by our
partner.

Lying on our side

Lying on the bed on our left side, possibly having our
upper leg supported either by a holder attached to the bed or
by our partner.

Birthing stool

Sitting on a stool with an opening in the front so the
baby has space to descend, and the nurse, midwife, or partner
can catch the baby.

Alternating walking and standing

Walking around and standing to let gravity help. It is very common to do what's called a "slow dance". For this, we will hold onto our partner and move our hips left and right as if we were slow dancing.

Lunging

Standing up, placing one of the legs on something higher, light a stool.

Forward leaning

It is like being on hands and knees but placing our arms on a higher surface like a yoga ball, or if we are on the bed, leaning over the back of the bed with many pillows on.

On hands and knees

Being in all four. This position allows for easy access to counter-pressure to alleviate discomfort.

Laying on our back

Not really recommended unless having an epidural. In this position, the coccyx forms what looks like a little mountain that the baby has to overcome to get out, making his exit a bit more difficult.

Pushing (2nd stage)

Spontaneous pushing

Pushing when our body feels the urge to push.

Laboring down

Holding for our skin and muscles around our pelvic area and perineum to be more flexible (to avoid tear) instead of starting pushing as soon as we are 10 centimeters dilated.

Directed pushing

Guided pushing by a nurse can be beneficial, especially if having an epidural and limited to no sensation in our legs.

Perineal care (2nd stage)

There are 4 degrees of perineum tear.

- First degree: It involves the skin and mucous membrane tearing. This one normally resolves on its own and it doesn't require repair after.
- Second degree: When also the perineal muscles tear. It might need a couple of stitches.
- Third degree: When also the anal sprinter tears. This is severe and it requires surgical repair.
- Fourth degree: When the rectal mucosa also tears. This is severe and it requires surgical repair.

Episiotomy/Prefer tear

An episiotomy is a deliberate cut made to the perineum to reduce the risk of tearing. However, tearing can still occur. We may choose to let a tear happen naturally. Normal tears are typically classified as degrees one or two.

Massage

Massaging the perineum can help the momentum of stretching and help avoid tears.

Warm compresses

Warm cloths applied to the perineum. Not hot, but warmed. This can be especially helpful in reducing 3-4 degree tears.

After delivery of the baby (3rd stage)

Catching the baby (mom, dad, doctor)

Marking our preference.

Cutting the umbilical cord (partner, doctor)

Depending on preference. These days it is more often for partners and dads to cut the cord.

Delayed cord clamping

Delaying cord clamping allows a few more pulses of

blood from the placenta to the newborn. This extra dose of blood can be as much as 30% - 40% of baby's blood volume.

The recommended delayed periods differ depending on the organization.

- The American College of Nurse-Midwives recommends 2-5 minutes.
- The WHO (World Health Organization) suggests 1-3 minutes.
- ACOG and AAP entrust 30-60 seconds, expressing special importance on delaying the clamping longer for preterm babies.

Cord blood donation

The option to donate our newborn's umbilical cord blood for use in life-saving transplantations or research. This is feasible if the hospital is part of a participating donation program, and we meet certain criteria, which are similar to the criteria for donating blood.

Cord blood saving for private banking

The option to bank our baby's cord blood for family use. If we are interested in this option, we would need to contact a private cord blood company. They will send us a kit that we would need to bring to the hospital for cord save keeping and pay the cost (monthly, yearly, or for life).

Delivery of the placenta (3rd stage)

The delivery of the placenta typically occurs with just a few more pushes. It often goes unnoticed because, at this point, our baby will likely already be resting on our chest. A midwife or nurse will provide assistance during this process.

Saving the placenta

The option to save the placenta and encapsulate it for consumption as a vitamin is controversial. Some believe the placenta, which is rich in nutrients and hormones, can offer various health benefits. However, the scientific community has not yet provided conclusive evidence supporting these claims.

Lotus Birth

This is a controversial one. It consists on leaving the cord attach to the placenta until it dries out.

- Positive point of view: it allows a full load transfer.
- Negative point of view: bacteria can colonize in the placenta and bring an infection.

Baby care (4th stage)

Skin-to-skin contact

Skin-to-skin normally happens right away after delivery and it's part of what's called the golden hour.

The golden hour: It involves spending the first hour of our baby's life with us, engaging in skin-to-skin contact.

> Skin-to-skin during the golden hour
> is a magical moment full of benefits
> for both mom and baby

Placing our baby on top of our skin is a powerful bonding experience. It is also very calming. It relaxes us and our baby. This action has many benefits, it stimulates baby's digestion and interest in feeding, and helps our milk production. It regulates baby's temperature, as well as baby's breathing and heart rate to better adapt to life outside of the womb. It also enables colonization of the baby's skin with our friendly bacteria which provides him/her with protection against infections.

Breastfeeding ASAP

Starting to give nutrients to our baby with our first milk (colostrum). Latching can be difficult at first, we can always consult a lactation expert. One may even come by our birthing room to provide help and advice.

Breastfeeding: It provides our baby with milk always at the perfect temperature, delivering essential antibodies they naturally received in the womb. This milk contains all the necessary nutrients, calories, and fluids crucial for our baby's health. It serves as a protective shield, guarding them against respiratory illnesses, diarrhea, and supporting their brain development and overall growth.

Colostrum: It is the initial milk we produce, a thick, sticky, yellowish liquid. The colostrum aids our baby's immune system by colonizing the gut with prebiotics and probiotics. Additionally, it creates a protective barrier against harmful bacteria, contributing to the overall well-being of our newborn.

Leave vernix on baby/Delay bath
The vernix is a viscose-like white substance that covers the baby. It protects the newborn's skin and facilitates extra-uterine adaptation of skin in the first postnatal week. Delaying the baby's first bath allows the vernix to be absorbed by the baby's skin.

Circumcision (if it is a boy)
If we have a boy, we can choose between have him circumcise or not. If choosing to circumcise, it's better to do so in the first or second day as the baby's skin is better for this procedure at this time. After that, anesthesia will be needed.

Erythromycin eye cream
It is used to prevent certain eye infections of newborn babies, like neonatal conjunctivitis, it is recommended to be given during the first 24h of birth.

Vitamin K
Vitamin K helps blood to clot. Babies are born with very small amounts of vitamin K in their bodies, this can lead

to bleeding problems. There are two options, oral vitamin K and the vitamins K shot. However, babies can't absorb the oral form very well.

Hepatitis B vaccine

It helps protect our baby from the Hepatitis B disease. By receiving the Hepatitis B vaccine, our baby is given a head start in building immunity against a viral infection that can potentially lead to liver-related complications.

Birth Plan Sample & Template

The power of having a place to start and use as a guide

Heather

BIRTH PLAN for _________________________________   MEDICAL #_________________

IN DELIVERY ROOM: *(partner)* _____________________   ***CONTACT:*** _______________

BABY'S NAME: _____________________   ***EDD:*** ___/___/202_   ***GENDER:*** ___________

Most important preferences

Natural unmedicated birth No medication offerings	Freedom of movement No episiotomy	Natural water rupture Skin to skin

Preferences for stage 1

LABOR

Interventions	Pain management	Relaxation techniques
None/Ask if emergency	Medication only offered if asked	Focused breathing
Hep lock only if required	Counter-pressure/Massages	Visualization
No IV	Hot/Cold packs	Walking/Changing positions
	Meditation/Exercises/Stretches	Hydrotherapy

Fetal Monitoring	Cervical Exams	Nutrition
Intermittent	Limited	Drinking
Handheld doppler	As needed	Eating
Being able to move		Ice chips/clear foods

Birth Environment

Limited people in room	Quiet voices
Dim lights	Music

Preferences for stage 2

PUSHING & DELIVERY

Birth Environment

Limited people in room	Quiet voices
Dim lights	Music

Labor and birth positions / *Pushing* / *Perineal Care*

Labor and birth positions	Pushing	Perineal Care
Hands and Knees	Spontaneous pushing	Prefer tear to episiotomy
Squatting	Labor down	Perineal Massage
Birth stool		Warm compresses
Side laying (peanut)		Slow crowning
Semi-sitting		

Preferences for stages 3 and 4

PLACENTA & BABY CARE

After Delivery	Golden Hour	Baby Care
Delayed cord clamping (45-60 sec or until slow pulsing)	Skin-to-skin contact	Hepatitis B vaccine
Ask partner about cutting cord	Breastfeeding asap	Vitamin K
NO circumcision	No bath for baby/Leave vernix	Erythromycin eye cream

<table>
<tr><td colspan="3" style="background:#ccc;">BIRTH PLAN for ___________________________   MEDICAL # ___________________</td></tr>
</table>

IN DELIVERY ROOM: *(partner)* _______________________   **CONTACT:** _______________

BABY'S NAME: ___________________   **EDD:** ___/___/202_   **GENDER:** _______________

MOST IMPORTANT PREFERENCES		
Natural unmedicated birth *No medication offerings*	*Freedom of movement* *No episiotomy*	*Natural water rupture* *Skin to skin*

STAGE 1 — LABOR

Interventions	Pain management	Relaxation techniques
None/Ask if emergency	Medication only offered if asked	Focused breathing
Hep lock only if required	Counter-pressure/Massages	Visualization
No IV	Hot/Cold packs	Walking/Changing positions
	Meditation/Exercises/Stretches	Hydrotherapy

Fetal Monitoring	Cervical Exams	Nutrition
Intermittent	Limited	Drinking
Handheld doppler	As needed	Eating
Being able to move		Ice chips/clear foods

Birth Environment	
Limited people in room	Quiet voices
Dim lights	Music

STAGE 2 — PUSHING & DELIVERY

Labor and birth positions	Pushing	Perineal Care
Hands and Knees	Spontaneous pushing	Prefer tear to episiotomy
Squatting	Labor down	Perineal Massage
Birth stool		Warm compresses
Side laying (peanut)		Slow crowning
Semi-sitting		

STAGE 3/4 — PLACENTA & BABY CARE

After Delivery	Golden Hour	Baby Care
Delayed cord clamping (45-60 sec or until slow pulsing)	Skin-to-skin contact	Hepatitis B vaccine
Ask partner about cutting cord	Breastfeeding asap	Vitamin K
NO circumcision	No bath for baby/Leave vernix	Erythromycin eye cream

Template

<table>
<tr><td colspan="3">BIRTH PLAN for ___________________________   MEDICAL #_________________</td></tr>
</table>

IN DELIVERY ROOM: (partner) _________________________   **CONTACT:** ______________

BABY'S NAME: ___________________   **EDD:** ___/___/202_   **GENDER:** ____________

MOST IMPORTANT PREFERENCES		
1.	2.	3.
4.	5.	6.

STAGE 1 — LABOR

Interventions	Pain management	Relaxation techniques

Fetal Monitoring	Cervical Exams	Nutrition

Birth Environment	

STAGE 2 — PUSHING & DELIVERY

Labor and birth positions	Pushing	Perineal Care

STAGE 3/4 — PLACENTA & BABY CARE

After Delivery	Golden Hour	Baby Care

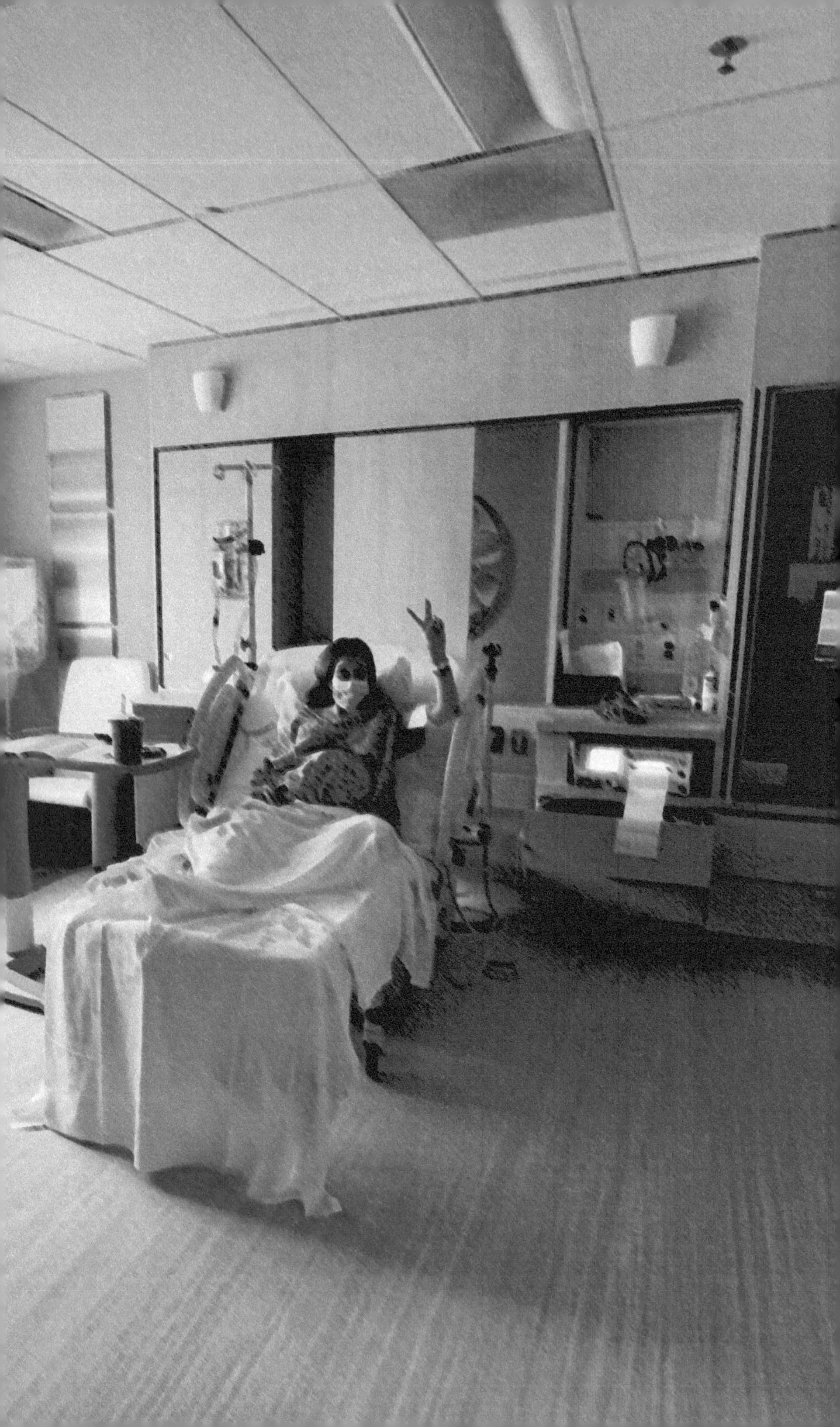

My Own Labor Experience

The power of embracing the unpredictable

I am a planner, though I know life dictates what happens in the labor room. My overall labor experience was good, and that's the answer I would give if someone asked. However, let's tell the whole truth.

Am I happy about my labor?
Yes.
How happy?
About 90%.
Is that a good number?
Sure.
Is that the percentage I would have love to say?
Not really.
Overall, would I describe my labor experience as positive?
Yes, I am glad to say that I had a positive birth experience.

Even before knowing I was pregnant, I debated between giving birth at a hospital, giving birth at a birthing clinic, and having a home birth.

Home-birth option

I considered a home birth early on, but it was discarded quite quickly. My bathtub is of standard size, and I didn't find it suitable for giving birth comfortably. While I thought about purchasing a birthing pool, and organizing all the necessary preparations, the idea of handling all these arrangements began to overwhelm me. The last thing I wanted during labor was to feel overwhelmed. I also felt some "social pressure" concerning the home setting, particularly in case complications arose. I have a blood condition that makes my blood thinner than usual, and I had placenta previa until the third trimester. Placenta previa is when the placenta is not on top of the uterus but below it and either occluding or almost occluding the opening of the vagina. Fortunately, my placenta moved out of the way by week 34. Until then, everything I had planned and wished for in my unmedicated vaginal delivery could potentially be pushed aside in favor of a cesarean birth. The thought of that happening was hard, but I remained resolute. I researched the acceptable distances between placenta and vagina to be able to make an informed decision if necessary; and, mainly, I focused on staying positive and I kept preparing my mind and body.

Birth clinic option

This time around, I went a different way. However, I am strongly considering it for my next birth, should I have another child. This time, insurance and financial considerations played a significant role in my decision.

Hospital option

I decided to have a natural birth in a hospital setting.

Before going into labor

I embraced my pregnancy, I believed in the power of my body and I was ready. I made sure to inform my provider about my desire for a natural birth and created a clear birth plan. I knew that during labor, my mind might be elsewhere, so I also ensured that my partner understood my priorities in case he needed to advocate for our birth plan.

Are these contractions?

Around 4 a.m., I woke up with a strange sensation in my belly. About 30 minutes later, I realized those sensations were contractions. At this point, I had slept for less than five hours, but I couldn't go back to sleep. I was so excited. My contractions had started, and it was real—it was happening. I can't recall if I woke up my husband or if he woke up because of my movements, but I do remember opening a contraction timer app on my phone, and together, we started timing the contractions. We chatted, happy to be experiencing this moment together, and time flew by.

Around 8 a.m., we began to prepare for the day. We both took showers, had breakfast, and double-checked that our hospital bag was ready and waiting by the door. The morning continued with contractions. They were occurring regularly but weren't quite long enough or close enough together. As time passed, the contractions became more intense, but I could manage them. We even managed to do some grocery shopping and take a walk while the contractions came and went. The only thing was that I needed to stop walking when the contractions peaked, but otherwise, I felt great. All the preparation was already being so very useful.

My water broke!

Around 1:30 p.m., I felt my water breaking. It wasn't a major gush, but liquid did come out. I still felt good, so I decided to have lunch. I knew that once in the hospital, I might not have the same freedom to make choices, like when to eat. As you'll read later, I'm glad I made that decision. Around 2:30-3 p.m., I called the hospital and I told them my *TACO* information. I told them I thought my water broke around 1:30p.m. (TIME), that there was not a lot (AMOUNT) and that it was clear (COLOR) with no smell (ODOR). I also let them know how I was in relation to the *5-1-1 rule*; I told them that I had contractions since 4:30 a.m. and that they were now about 5 minutes apart, lasting for 1 minute every time. I asked them if it was time to head over there—I really did not want to arrive at the hospital and be sent back. They replied "yes" so I went ahead.

Checking-in at the hospital

I arrived soon after, and at 4 p.m. I was admitted into the hospital. The funny part was that when I was checking into the hospital, they asked me if I was the one who had called ahead of time. Perhaps nobody usually calls in advance? They explained it was partly because of that, and partly because there was only one other woman in the hospital that day. It turned out to be a surprisingly quiet day.

Now, let's discuss what happened before I was officially admitted as an inpatient. They provided me with a hospital gown and disposable underwear, and walked me to a small room. They asked me numerous questions, drew my blood, and monitored the baby's and my heart rate for 10-20 minutes. One of the questions they kept asking was how much pain I was having from 0 (none) to 10 (excruciating), I did not enjoy that this question focused on the pain, but it was standard practice. The nurse was very kind, treating me with respect and attentiveness. I explained my intention for an unmedicated birth, and she understood.

I was thrilled that I arrived at the hospital during the day because, in my hospital, there are two doctors during the day and two at night, but only one midwife, and only during the day. So there I was, waiting to see if I would be admitted.

When the nurse informed me I was in, and the midwife
would assist me, I was overjoyed. Not only was it daytime,
but I was lucky they had assigned the midwife to assist me in
my birth. I was very excited because I believed the midwife
would approach the birth more holistically and have a deeper
understanding of a natural birth. However, all the luck and
happiness I was feeling vanished as soon as I met her. Very
unfortunate.

Meeting the Midwife

She entered the room and right away initiated an
abrupt conversation:
- Midwife: "So you have no pain now, huh? What are
  you going to do when you feel pain?"
- Me: "I plan to cope with pain through meditation
  and..."
- Midwife (interrupting): "This is not a walk in the
  park."
- Me: "I know."
- Midwife: "Is this your first child?"
- Me: "Yes."
- Midwife (laughs as if to suggest I don't know
  anything because it's my first child): "Have you
  taken any classes?"
- Me: "Yes, I attended classes, read books, and did
  various exercises in preparation."

That was not at all how I expected to be treated (by
the midwife, or any health professional for that matter).
The skepticism and the disrespect were not how I wanted to
start my birth experience, but there is only so much one can
control. Especially after I had decided I would deliver in the
hospital and that was it, the day of the delivery of my baby
boy.

After the brief conversation with the midwife, she

proceeded to perform a cervical exam to check if my water had indeed broken and how many centimeters I was dilated. While checking my dilation, anything but gently, she was making faces and saying numbers to the nurse. It was like if I was not there, I did not need to know what all those numbers and specific terms were but I am someone who values being informed, besides no informed decision can ever be made without having the necessary information.

I asked a few questions in an attempt to get a better understanding of what was happening, it was my body being discussed after all. She confirmed that I was one centimeter dilated, that my membranes had ruptured in a somewhat uncommon place, higher than usual, and that the baby's head was blocking the hole, which explained why only a small amount of liquid had come out. Following a few tests, I was officially admitted to the hospital.

The delivery room

At this point, about 12 hours had passed since my contractions had started. I was transferred to a comfortable delivery room that had everything needed for childbirth, including a couch that could transform into a bed for my husband, should we spend the night there, which we did. I asked my husband to bring the hospital bags from the car.

Once we settled, we chatted like it was a normal day, the only difference being that when a contraction would arrive, I would get into a squat position or I would get on my hands and knees to ease the intensity of the contractions.

Is anyone looking at my birth plan?

I brought three birth plan copies. I gave the first one to the first nurse, then that copy got lost, so I gave the copy I got for myself to the next nurse. I told my husband to hold onto third copy should we needed it again. We also had a copy in our phone, but during labor the phone was the last thing we were thinking about—although, we did use it to take a few memorable pictures, and to put my birthing playlists and create a nice environment.

At 7 p.m., the nursing shift changed. I got to meet my night nurse, who, while nice, was not as friendly as the daytime nurse. Around 30 minutes later, the new nurse brought some pain medications for me (I wasn't experiencing pain, and I had no intention of taking unnecessary medication). I reminded her about my preference for an unmedicated birth. However, it became evident through several moments during the night that they might not have reviewed my birth plan.

I said, "no, thank you!"

Soon after, the midwife entered the room and indicated that they were going to administer Pitocin. I declined, which the midwife did not appreciate. With a so no great attitude she expressed the need to induce labor because I wasn't progressing, citing my low pain level as a reason. They didn't perform additional cervical exams; the assumption was that my lack of pain meant slow progress. I explained that I might have a higher pain tolerance, sharing that I had experienced a broken bone without excruciating pain.

After some back and forth, I insisted we wait. As our conversation was ending, my baby boy moved his head, and the amniotic fluid, which had not flowed earlier when my water broke, suddenly gushed out, creating a big puddle on the floor. The midwife looked at floor and then looked at me and rolled her eyes.

About an hour later, more intense contractions began, but it would take several hours to reach the pushing stage. Reaching 10 centimeters dilation was challenging; I had many contractions, but my dilation progressed slowly. I believe the negative environment, critical comments, and judgmental expressions from the medical team contributed to the prolonged labor. Fortunately, the midwife's shift ended at 11 p.m., and I was assigned a doctor. This doctor was much kinder and respectful.

Oh well, I did not expect that...

As the night passed, I was getting more and more tired. I had only slept 4-5 hours the night before, and I hadn't eaten anything since lunch, so I was glad I had eaten when I did. The night took a turn when baby shifted and was pressing on my sciatic nerve, that actually was painful. I was fine with the discomfort of the contractions, but both of my legs aching and constantly shaking took me by surprise.

My husband was a caring and encouraging presence, reminding me of the various exercises and techniques we had practiced before the birth to cope with the pain; the breathing, the changing positions, the vocalizations, etc. In the early morning, I would pass out in between contractions, and having him by my side, encouraging me with meditation and breathing exercises, especially the ocean visualization, was incredibly helpful.

Unexpected developments

Moving and changing positions was working fantastically until I started to have too many contractions every time I moved. At one point, I needed to use the bathroom and, if I remember correctly, that led to six contractions in less than three minutes. This stressed the baby as he did not have time enough to recover in between contractions. I was pulled from the bathroom, placed on the bed, attached to monitors, and given an oxygen mask. In that moment, baby was not ok. The priority was to restore the baby's heart rate and my blood oxygen levels to normal.

My hep-lock for emergencies became handy. They connected me to an IV for a saline solution. I understand they needed to act fast, but I also wish there had been better communication. Even though, both the mask and the saline solution were used only for a short period of time, I felt left in the dark. If the mask and the saline solution were necessary, I would have consented to them regardless. I denied unnecessary medications (some random pills they were trying to give me, the Pitocin, the epidural, etc), but if something was imperative to ensure my baby's and my health, I understand and I am grateful for it.

Sadly, the nurses' actions at this point were not in line with my birth plan or personal preferences, which made me feel undervalued and uninformed. I felt discouraged but as I planned, I did not let this situation determine the course of the night. I breathed in and out, and accepted what happened and how it happened so that I could keep myself going in a positive mindset.

Salt water and oxygen were the most natural way they could proceed I was told later on.

Thank goodness I persevered

After this incident, I was not allowed to move out of the bed. Lying on my back was exactly what I did not want and I had to advocate for myself. Then they said I could move as long as I stayed on the bed. Moving side to side was like magic. It was not perfect, but just that felt so good.

Some contractions were easier to deal with than others. The nurse repeatedly asked me if I wanted an epidural. I lost count of how many times I refused it, emphasizing that they should not ask me again. I vividly remember some of her comments and questions:

- "Are you sure you don't want the epidural?"
- "You look like you are in so much pain..."

- "I am not sure if you are going to be able to do this."
- "The epidural would help you."
- "You don't have to be a hero, you know?"
- "Don't be a martyr."
- You are running out of time to get the epidural, you should get it now."

This was not part of my birth plan. I had specifically mentioned that medications should only be offered if I requested them. To be honest, after the constant insistence, there was a moment when I even doubted my ability to deliver my son. Luckily, I found the strength to persevere, thanks to all the preparation during the pregnancy, my husband's support, and the use of affirmations. Thank goodness.

An angel appeared...

The night improved when my nurse needed to go on break and a different nurse came to cover for her. This new nurse was a true angel. She quickly noticed that I was very uncomfortable and, in a split second, brought six pillows, placing three on each side of me to support my shaking legs, and gave me some heat packs. This significantly eased the terrible leg pain. Then, she helped with some new breathing exercises and promoted a more relaxing atmosphere. Unfortunately, I didn't have the chance to learn her name, but she made a remarkable impact.

Time to push

When I reached 10 centimeters and could begin pushing, I felt great. Pushing itself didn't hurt, it was the holding stage before reaching 10 centimeters that had been challenging. I had felt the urge to push for a while, and I was ready. I cannot recall how long the pushing stage lasted;

my husband estimates it was about an hour, it felt faster for me. The time it took did not matter and, in fact, the slow and steady crowning was worth it. I felt no pain, only the sensation known as the "ring of fire," which was manageable, and I had zero tears.

"Open your eyes, now!"

For various reasons, I kept my eyes closed for most of my labor; I was tired, wanted to avoid judgmental looks, and aimed to create my own tranquil environment.

At 5:41 a.m., the doctor said in a firm voice, "Open your eyes now." I opened them and, just like in that famous children's lion movie, I witnessed my baby boy rising up. My beautiful son was here with us. The nurse padded him clean a little and placed him on my chest. While I was captivated by him, the doctor and nurses attended to the delivery of the placenta and ensured everything was in order.

They were amazed that I had delivered without an epidural, felt nothing during the placenta extraction, and were especially surprised that I had no tears.

Grateful

With all these, I want to thank my old self for going through the preparation process. The effort, practice, and readiness enabled me to have a birth experience I do not regret. It was not perfect and it had moments that were not as I planned, but I was able to give birth to my son naturally without any tears, which facilitated a speedy recovery. A couple days later I was feeling myself again.

The best part is that now I not only have the prep but the experience itself. I know what I would keep, what I would change, and when I would be more assertive to make my next labor even better.

About the Author

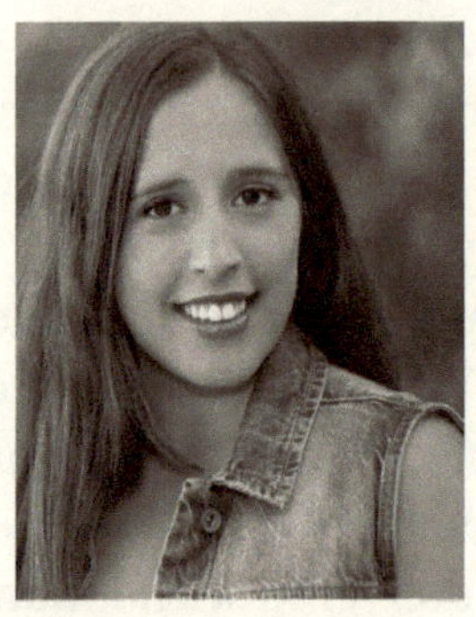

Sandra Lena is a dynamic and multifaceted professional from Spain currently based in Los Angeles, CA. From an early age, Sandra was driven by a desire to inspire and uplift others. She holds degrees in Audiovisual media and Journalism, and is a fitness instructor certified in prenatal and postnatal training. Sandra's global journey has enriched her craft, allowing her to merge fitness, and storytelling with a unique cultural lens. As an author, Sandra's literary debut *Historias de Comienzo,* became an best-seller remaining on top charts for weeks. Later, expanding her creative footprint by delving into the world of children's books, she created the bilingual series *Abby the Bee,* where her imaginative storytelling intertwines with an engaging learning experience for young readers in both English and Spanish. In film and TV, Sandra is an International Award-Winning video editor and filmmaker. Her multidisciplinary background shapes every project she touches, bringing a distinct creative signature rooted in passion.